21 Days to a Joy-Filled Life

21 Days to a Joy-Filled Life

*The Donut Dare - Focus on All You Have,
Not All That's Missing*

Vicki Huffman

Printed by CreateSpace, An Amazon.com Company

21 Days to a Joy-Filled Life

This book is intended as a resource only. Any information provided here is designed to assist you in making informed decisions about your health. It is not intended to replace the advice of, or treatment prescribed by, a medical professional. If you suspect you may have a medical problem, seek out competent medical assistance.

Any Internet addresses (websites, blogs, etc.) referenced in this book are offered as a resource. Mention of specific companies, organizations or authorities does not imply endorsement of this book. Internet addresses were accurate at the time this book went to print.

Book Design by Vicki Huffman

Author Photo by Stephani Bush

Scripture quotations marked (NLT) are taken from the Holy Bible, New Living Translation, copyright © 1996, 2004, 2007 by Tyndale House Foundation. Used by permission of Tyndale House Publishers, Inc., Carol Stream, Illinois 60188. All rights reserved

Scripture quotations marked (TLB) are taken from The Living Bible, copyright © 1971. Used by permission of Tyndale House Publishers, Inc., Wheaton, IL 60189. All rights reserved.

Printed in the United States of America

First printing June, 2017

Contents

Getting Started 1

Day 1: Count Your Blessings 5

Day 2: How Food Affects Your Mood 11

Day 3: Ask for Help 17

Day 4: Dispute Negative Thoughts 23

Day 5: Have Faith 31

Day 6: Get Up and Move 37

Day 7: Practice Enjoying Life 41

Day 8: Master Your Mind and Habits 47

Day 9: Remember Happy Times 55

Day 10: Practice Prayer and Meditation 61

Day 11: Create Wellness Habits 67

Day 12: Identify Your Triggers 73

Day 13: Learn About Depression 77

Day 14: Get Your Sleep 83

Day 15: Be Spontaneous 89

Day 16: Energize Yourself 93

Day 17: Increase Your Face-Time 97

Day 18: Explore New Interests 101

Day 19: Help Others 105

Day 20: Enhance Your Spiritual Life...109

Day 21: Pick Your Battles 113

Documenting Your Journey..119

Notes...223

Who Am I 227

Getting Started

What is the Donut Dare?

The Donut Dare has nothing to do with food and everything to do with learning to enjoy the goodness around you. It requires you to stop focusing on what's missing in your life, the donut hole, and focus on all you have, the donut. Simply put, stop focusing on what's wrong and focus on what's right!

The Donut Dare is a 21-day challenge to change the way you think and act by focusing only on what is good and right. It's a task that will require:

- An all-in commitment

- Continuous self-examination

- Action followed by reflection

This is a personal journey. It is a guided tour to your joy-filled life. The amount of effort you put in will determine your success on this journey and whether you reach the finish line. I know you can make it. Just follow in my footsteps. You may need to stop along the way and spend a little more time on something, and that's okay. The goal is to finish strong not to be the first one there.

> Joy: *a deep feeling* or *condition* of *happiness* or *contentment.*[1]

The Return of Joy

Joy is a condition many seek but few find. Today you are starting a journey which will take you there. I will be with you every step of the way as your personal tour guide. Why? Because I've taken this journey many times and always managed to end up back where I started. Until now.

A few years back, I suffered an emotional breakdown following 40 years with depression. That's when I said, "Never Again!" I committed to finding out how to live a life filled with joy. So over the next 21 days you will follow my footsteps. With dedication and hard work, you too can experience a joy-filled life.

What Will the Next 21 Days Look Like?

Each day will be structured the same. We will start by exploring the focus for the day, followed by three activities:

- *Process* what you've learned about the focus idea presented

- *Engage* in an activity designed to implement the new skills

- *Reflect* on the new skills, and plan to use them regularly

You'll read the focus idea and do your *Process* journaling early in the day. Then complete the *Engage* activities throughout the day, and finish up with the *Reflect* journaling activity. Let's look at each in more detail.

Process

Let the new idea or skill sink in. The questions will check for understanding. Resources are listed for further study. (*Links have been shortened using bitly.com*)

Use the journal at the back of this book to assess yourself and record your thoughts about the daily topic.

Engage

This is where the work happens. It's time to implement what you discovered about yourself in the focus area. It may require you to create something or physically do something. But don't worry, it's nothing difficult.

If you need more than one day to implement the new skill, you have two choices.

- Option A – Continue through the full 21-day journey as an overview. Then, return to areas where you need more time for reinforcement or reflection. This allows exposure to all the ideas and skills in 21 days. You may not master all of them, but who knows, the one thing you really need may be on Day 20.

- Option B – Quit counting the days, and stay on a skill until you master it. I'd rather you take 60 days than give up because it's not working. This allows you to master each skill before moving on.

These skills will become habits. But you need to practice them every day for the remainder of the journey to ensure your joyful success.

Use the journal at the back of this book to complete the activities on the worksheets I've provided. Want to be more creative? Get your own journal and make it personal.

Reflect

Think about how things went for the day. What went right? What didn't? What would you do differently next time? How did you feel?

Use the journal at the back of this book to plan how you will embed the new skill into your life on a regular basis.

Why Do I Have to Write It All Down?

You may not enjoy journaling. I didn't. When they handed me a notebook in the hospital and told me to write in it, I had flashbacks of my *Dear Diary* days. If you're feeling the same way, you may not understand the importance of documenting your journey.

What would we do if previous generations hadn't documented their journey through life? History, even our own, is powerful. It reminds us of things we enjoyed or did well. It also teaches us things to avoid, shows us how far we've come, and what we've learned.

Just try it. Don't worry; it gets easier. Writing things down forces you to think a little deeper. Because you must understand before you can explain. A slower pace also ensures you don't leave anything out.

The Journal focuses on five areas of strength:

- Mental Wellness

- Physical Wellness

- Spiritual Wellness

- Emotional Wellness

- Wellness Action Plan

Strength in these five areas is needed to live the joy-filled life. You may only need help in one or two areas. You may need help in all five. Whatever your situation, help is ahead.

I Think I'm Ready

How many times have you said, "I can't take it anymore; something's got to change?" Let this be the last. Do you want to enjoy life again? Are you up for the challenge? I dare you. I Donut Dare you! If you're ready, open your heart to the sweet joy of life, and join me on the journey to a joy-filled life.

Day 1: Count Your Blessings

How was my day? Well, I lost my job, my son got suspended for fighting, and my dog threw up on the carpet. It won't take long to count my blessings – I don't have any!

Ever feel like this? You have nothing for which to be thankful? Look again. You are focusing on what's missing in your life, instead of what you have. It's time to change your focus. It's time for a donut dare!

Let's start our journey by recognizing everyone feels like this at some point. However, if you take an honest look at your life, you'll realize you have a lot to be thankful for. Just watch the news for five minutes and you'll start counting your blessings. Let's list a few you may have forgotten:

- A Roof Over Your Head (even if it's not your own, you're probably not sleeping on the ground outside exposed to the elements)

- Clean Water (even if it's not bottled or filtered, you're probably not having to cup your hands in a dirty river to get drinking water)

- Hot Meals (even if they're provided by a shelter, hospital, assisted living facility, or jail)

- Indoor Plumbing (or an outhouse for that matter – somewhere set aside for this specific purpose, you're probably not squatting behind a tree)

- Access to knowledge and education (whether it be at a school, on the Internet, TV, newspapers, books you own or at a public library)

- Shoes (something not made from a flattened 2-liter bottle with a rope strap fashioned into a flip flop – yes, I've seen a child wearing this)

Is that enough to help you start focusing on all you have? People all over the world lack these simple pleasures. They would give anything to have a job to lose, a child to get suspended, or a dog, even if it threw up.

Yes, you may have had a rotten day. But in the whole scheme of things, you've still got it pretty good.

So let's examine that a little further. What's the difference between a want and a need? A need is something you require because it is essential or very important.[1] A want, on the other hand, is something you desire to possess or do. You wish for it.[2] You may find you want much more than you actually need.

Make a list of what you need (remember that means require) to get through the day? Keep in mind, you need food, but you want steak. You need water, but you want something from a bottle or through a filter. You need shelter, but you want a home of your own. You need clothing, but you want name brands. You need transportation, but you want your own vehicle.

Now refine your list until it includes only basic needs (ie. food, water, shelter, etc). I think this is a good time to look at that word – contentment – from our definition earlier. It means being mentally or emotionally satisfied with things as they are.[3] That's our goal – Learning to be content with what we have. Enjoying the donut without missing or desiring the hole.

Process *(remember to head to the journal in the back of the book for this)*

Have you ever thought about how many things you have which others around the world don't? Have you ever visited a homeless shelter or a food pantry? Each of us has people nearby without many of the simple comforts we take for granted. How can you make yourself more aware of those in your community who go without these things?

Engage *(remember to head to the journal in the back of the book for this)*

Create a Blessings Box. Find an old shoe box, or plastic container with a lid. Decorate it if you'd like. Make it something you enjoy having around. Not creative? You can buy a beautiful box at any hobby store. Next, get some paper, either plain or colored, and some colorful pencils or markers.

Cut a sheet of paper into about six pieces. They can be strips, circles, triangles or squares; the shape doesn't matter. Have fun with it. On each piece, write something you are blessed to have. I gave you some above, so start with those if you'd like, but be specific.

Hopefully, you thought of others. Cut another sheet. Or two. Think of as many blessings as you can. Remember to go beyond your basic needs to see your blessings. Think outside the box. Include friends, something in nature you enjoy, good health, and eyesight to name just a few. Believe me, you have no clue how valuable good health is until you're with someone who doesn't have it.

Set the Blessings Box somewhere you can see it frequently. As you go through the 21 days, add to it. If you are having a rough day, like the one described earlier, dump out and explore your Blessings Box. Count your blessings. Think about them one by one. Then think about what life would be like without them. You'll feel more joyful in no time.

Be Inspired. Start a new habit of being inspired daily. Take time to read scripture, a devotional, or an inspirational book. Listen to uplifting music, and focus on the lyrics. Digest their meaning and how they inspire you. According to David Niven, author of *The 100 Simple Secrets of Happy People*, music can have a positive effect on mood in 92% of people.[4] Try it out. It can't hurt.

I will list a few Inspiration Suggestions each day. Pick one or two, and think about them throughout the day. Let them sink into your heart and mind.

Inspiration Suggestions

> *Better to lose count while naming your blessings than to lose your blessings to counting your troubles. Maltbie D. Babcock*
>
> *Let all that I am praise the Lord; may I never forget the good things he does for me. Psalms 103:2 (NLT)*
>
> *Song – Blessings by Laura Story**
>
> *Song – This is the Stuff by Francesca Battistelli**
>
> *Song – Day One by Matthew West**
>
> **Video available at https://sadnesstojoy.com/inspiration/music*

Reflect *(remember to head to the journal in the back of the book for this)*

1. What did you think, talk, and post about today? Were you able to stay focused on the donut (your blessings, what's going right), or did you spend the day focused on the hole (your misfortune, what's going wrong)?

2. What will you need to do to learn to be content with what you have?

3. How will you implement what you discovered today to help you find joy?

4. What did you feel when you thought about the homeless near you who have so little? What did you learn through this exercise?

5. Were you able to draw a clear line between wants and needs? How did it make you feel to realize so many things you thought were needs are really wants?

6. How many blessings were you able to add to your box? What were your thoughts when you realized how truly blessed you were?

7. Which of the Inspiration Suggestions did you choose? What stood out that you'd like to remember?

8. Go to https://sadnesstojoy.com/forum/21days, and share your thoughts about counting your blessings.

Day 2: How Food Affects Your Mood

You came back for Day 2! That makes you a winner already. This is not an easy journey, and I'm glad you didn't quit when you realized that. I'm also glad we are going to continue to walk it together, so I can help point out some of the pitfalls since I've already been down this road before. Today let me guide you through an understanding of how food affects your mood.

Ice cream. Birthday cake. Cheetos®. Chocolate. What do these foods have in common? They are my favorite comfort foods; the foods I turn to when I'm feeling emotional. Also, they hold very little, if any, nutritional value.

Multiple studies point out the importance of a healthy diet. Eat your fruits and vegetables. Drink plenty of water. Consume whole-grains. These are a few universal agreements. Fats in moderation is universal, but what constitutes a healthy fat is difficult to decipher. Plant- or animal-based proteins is a matter of choice, but eating protein is universal.

Those were the *Do's*. Now, for the *Don'ts*. Avoid alcohol, caffeine, sugar, and refined carbs. What in the world is a refined carb? Not all carbohydrates are the same. All sugars and starches, except those that come in the form of a natural whole food like a piece of fruit or a sweet potato, are considered refined carbohydrates.[1]

The Centers for Disease Control and Prevention (CDC) reports 20.8% of adults in America eat less than one vegetable every day. The statistic is even more alarming in adolescents, with 40.2% eating less than one vegetable a day.[2]

Most of us know what we need to eat, but we allow our emotions to guide our food choices. When we aren't feeling well, we reach for what makes us feel better or what's easy to grab. That's usually processed foods with very little nutrition. A better choice would be foods high in Vitamin B, Vitamin D, and Omega-3 Fatty Acids. These foods boost your mood, so consume plenty of them. Head to my website at https://sadnesstojoy.com/resources/help-for-depression/#food-affects-mood, or my Pinterest page at http://pinterest.com/vickihuffman23 to find some healthy options.

Our bodies, and our emotions, function best when they are provided with the nutrients needed. Let's look at a car and how fuel affects its performance. My daughter owned a car which required diesel fuel. She had to go out of her way on many occasions to locate a gas station which had diesel fuel. It was a huge inconvenience, but she did it. Why? Because if she put regular fuel in her diesel tank, the car would stop working.

Our bodies are the same. If we don't put the proper fuel in our body, disease will slow us down. If we continue feeding our body the wrong fuel, it will eventually shut down, just like that car.

If you are trying to eat healthier, the easiest tip to remember when shopping for food is to focus primarily on the outer perimeter of the grocery store. Most fresh fruits, vegetables, dairy products, meats, and natural foods are usually located on the outer aisles.[3]

Also remember to eat foods in their most natural state. For instance, eat an orange rather than orange juice. Another tip is to find food with the least number of ingredients. For example, fresh or frozen foods are always better than canned.

I'm not a nutritionist, so I rely on the experts to help me find a healthy diet that meets my tastes and lifestyle. Check out these links located on my website at https://sadnesstojoy.com/resources/help-for-depression/#how-food-affects-mood.

- Dietary Guidelines for Americans 2015-2020 – http://bit.ly/2fqJsNN

- Diagnosis: Diet – Psychology Today – http://bit.ly/2cxUsHh

- Nutrition – CDC - http://bit.ly/2elyx7W

- SuperTracker – USDA – http://bit.ly/2coLst1

- Improving Your Emotional Health Through Healthier Eating – Psych Central – http://bit.ly/2eGjuc3

- Healthy Eating – Help Guide – http://bit.ly/1tqLrqK

- *Made to Crave* by Lysa TerKeurst – http://bit.ly/2nrKkW2

Process

What did you learn about healthy eating? Learning to eat healthy is a process. Knowledge is the first step. Next is implementation.

Were you aware your dietary choices could be affecting how you feel emotionally? The food you eat could be affecting your level of joy. Dr. Joseph Mercola says, "Whether you need a quick pick-me-up or you've been struggling with poor mood for a while, the best place to start to turn your mood around is likely not in your medicine cabinet but right in your pantry or refrigerator."[4]

Engage

After reviewing the links provided above, plan a healthier diet.

Create a Meal Plan. Get a monthly or weekly calendar, or use the blank Meal Plan provided. Use the planning tools from the *SuperTracker* link above to start filling in your calendar. Start with just one week. Don't forget to allow for leftovers. For instance, plan a second meal with leftover baked chicken such as chicken soup, chicken salad or a chicken casserole. There are loads of recipes online. Pinterest is my go-to site.

Use a Food Tracker. The *SuperTracker* link above is a good one. If you prefer something on your smart phone for portability, I use Under Armour's *MyFitnessPal* app.[5] You can select from basic foods, restaurant menu items or create your own item, where it calculates the nutrition information based on the recipe you enter.

Track what you eat every day, and yes, you do have to include everything you consume, including drinks, candy, gum and mints. Seeing how much sugar I was consuming daily was a real shocker. I found it helpful to check my intake right before dinner. This allowed me to alter my plan if necessary to better meet my daily goals.

Be Inspired. Take time to read scripture, a devotional, or an inspirational book. Listen to uplifting music, and focus on the lyrics. Digest their meaning and how they inspire you.

Inspiration Suggestions

The doctor of the future will give no medication but will interest his patients in the care of the human frame, diet, and in the cause and prevention of disease. Thomas A. Edison

Let food be thy medicine, thy medicine shall be thy food. Hippocrates

One should eat to live, not live to eat. Benjamin Franklin

Please eat something now for your own good. Acts 27:34a (NLT)

Reflect

1. What did you think, talk, and post about today? Were you able to stay focused on the donut (the many healthy food choices you can eat), or did you spend the day focused on the hole (all the food choices you shouldn't eat, including actual donuts)?

2. How will you implement what you discovered today to help you find joy?

3. What did you learn about healthy eating? What improvements could you make to your current eating habits?

4. What changes are necessary based on your food tracking? What will you do differently?

5. What obstacles will you need to overcome to follow healthier eating habits? How will you overcome them?

6. Which of the Inspiration Suggestions did you choose? What stood out that you'd like to remember?

7. Go to https://sadnesstojoy.com/forum/21days, and share your thoughts about how food affects your mood.

Day 3: Ask for Help

I know it's not easy to give up your favorite foods. Remember – I've already walked this road. If you love food as much as I do, I'm impressed you came back for Day 3. I promise it's worth it, because dietary changes will make things better. So stick with it. Now, let me meddle a little further. It's time to recognize this journey was not meant to be traveled alone, so let's learn to ask for help.

─────────────

"I do it myself," is the cry of every two-year old. Independence is something we learn at a very early age. It is a good thing to learn. However, we can take it too far. Are you an independence addict? I was.

Asking for help is one of the hardest things adults encounter, since it is often viewed as a weakness. For instance, my 82-year old mother refuses to allow me to carry her bag through the airport even though carrying it completely wears her out. She doesn't want to admit she can't do something, to be a burden, appear needy, or look like she doesn't have it all together. But the truth is, we all need help at different times in our life.

When it comes to your health, whether physical, mental, emotional, or spiritual, people are generally all too willing to help where they can. If family and friends knew you were struggling, they might even offer to help without you having to ask.

Let's put it in perspective. If you found a lump, had trouble breathing, or had severe headaches, you most likely wouldn't hesitate to ask for help. That's why doctors exist. To diagnose disease, and manage your symptoms. These are all physical in nature, but what about mental or emotional symptoms?

There are several types of medical professionals available to assist with these concerns as well. Psychiatrists are medical doctors who specialize in the diagnosis and treatment of mental illness. They are the only mental health professionals licensed to prescribe medication for illnesses such as depression or anxiety.

Closely related, from a patient perspective, are the Psychotherapist (Therapist) and the Psychologist. They are both non-medical professionals who specialize in the science side of human behavior. They provide treatment of mental illness through individual and group behavioral therapy. In other words, they help you change the way you see things and any habits associated with these distorted views.

Now the decision to seek medical assistance is a personal one. Not everyone wants to withstand the stigma associated with it. The cost, especially without insurance, is often prohibitive as well. That's fine. It may not be for you. However, help is still out there.

Your pastor or spiritual advisor is a non-medical professional who is trained in counseling. If you don't attend a local church, stop by during the day to meet the pastor. If he can't help you personally, he will be able to recommend someone who can.

Another option is a friend or family member. They're available anytime and are free of charge, but seek out someone you trust to keep your discussions private. Your best candidate is someone compassionate and caring but firm enough to hold you accountable for change.

If you've given up hope of ever getting better, or don't want to try anymore, immediately contact your local mental health professional, employee assistance helpline, or the Suicide Prevention Lifeline at 1-800-273-TALK (8255).

The first step toward wellness is to ask for help. Mental health wellness requires a strong commitment, hard work, and people who support you. But it can be done. You can feel better!

Process

What were your thoughts when I asked if you were an independence addict? Do you have a hard time asking for help? The following links are some of my favorite sites which clarify mental health professionals' roles, what help is available, how you can find it, and some self-help resources.

- National Alliance on Mental Illness (NAMI) – http://bit.ly/V1KdCa

- National Institute of Mental Health (NIH) – http://bit.ly/2eTPLNe

- Anxiety & Depression Association of America (ADAA) – http://bit.ly/2ddCwlV

- Suicide Prevention Lifeline – http://bit.ly/1lYmABO

- Sadness to Joy – https://sadnesstojoy.com/resources/help-for-depression

Engage

After reviewing the links provided above, decide who might be the best person to help you at this point in your life. It may be a professional. It may be a family member or friend. Only you can decide.

Make an Appointment. After you have decided who will provide the help and support you need, make an appointment to meet with them. If you contact a mental health professional's office, you can often wait a month or more for an appointment. If you need help sooner, say so. If they are unable to accommodate your need, ask to be placed on a cancellation waiting list or contact another provider. Help finding a local provider is available through the links above.

If you've decided to seek help from a friend, let them know why you want to meet with them. Set a time and place most comfortable and convenient for you, not them. It should be somewhere private, as emotions will most likely be strong.

Be Inspired. Take time to read scripture, a devotional, or an inspirational book. Listen to uplifting music, and focus on the lyrics. Digest their meaning and how they inspire you.

Inspiration Suggestions

With self-discipline, most anything is possible. Theodore Roosevelt

Suffer the pain of discipline, or suffer the pain of regret. Jim Rohn

Weeping may last through the night, but joy comes with the morning. Psalm 30:5 (NLT)

Song – Hope in Front of Me by Danny Gokey*

Song – Need You Now (How Many Times) by Plumb*

*Video available at https://sadnesstojoy.com/inspiration/music

Author's Note: I probably listened to these two songs about a dozen times each during the first few weeks of my mental wellness recovery journey. I found them to be quite inspirational. They brought me hope and reminded me no matter how far down I had fallen, there were better days ahead. I knew I couldn't do it on my own. But I also knew I wasn't alone.

Reflect

1. What did you think, talk, and post about today? Were you able to stay focused on the donut (help is available to you), or did you spend the day focused on the hole (you're all alone and no one understands)?

2. How will you implement what you discovered today to help you find joy?

3. Do you want to feel better, even if it means hard work and talking about how you got to where you are today? Are you willing to explore why you feel the way you do, even if it means digging into your past?

4. How does the term Mental Illness make you feel? Can you live with the stigma?

5. Which of the Inspiration Suggestions did you choose? What stood out that you'd like to remember?

6. Go to https://sadnesstojoy.com/forum/21days, and share your thoughts about asking for help.

Day 4: Dispute Negative Thoughts

Yesterday, we learned to admit we need help. To acknowledge we may not be telling ourselves the truth when we say no one will understand. No one wants to be bothered. It's time to take the next step on our journey and acknowledge that every thought that enters our mind is not true.

We may be the victim of our own bullying. Bullies attempt to humiliate us, belittle us, and make us feel hopeless and alone. Sometimes our mind creates and lingers on thoughts designed to do the same thing. I'm not going to lie to you, this part of our journey is rather difficult. So the best way to get through it is to take my hand and step exactly in my footsteps. I got through it. You can too. Let's go.

_____

She makes me so angry.

I feel so stupid when he talks to me that way.

I'm such a loser.

There are many technical names for these types of statements, like cognitive distortion or automatic thoughts. But I just call them negative thoughts. They pop into your mind without any warning and tend to linger there. In most cases, these negative thoughts are lies. Works of fiction which are not to be believed. In this way, they are like the hurtful words of a bully. They are meant to get inside our head and make us question our worth.

William Shakespeare said, "There is nothing either good or bad, but thinking makes it so." Eleanor Roosevelt said it another way, "No one can make you feel inferior without your consent." The point they share is this – when something happens, you can choose how you look at it. Is it an obstacle or an opportunity? However, when emotions are involved, that choice doesn't seem so clear. It may require some effort, but how you view it is still your choice.

All of us have negative thoughts at times. Some handle them better than others. What's the trick? Learning to distinguish fact from fiction. Just because we feel something, or think something, doesn't mean it's true. That's why jurors are directed to examine the evidence, not their feelings about the evidence. It's important to do the same with our thoughts.

But examining the evidence behind our thoughts requires us to slow down and be more aware of them or reflect on them later. We'll learn more about awareness on Day 8, but for now, just reflect on your thoughts at the end of each day.

What thoughts and feelings are you having that you can't seem to get out of your mind? Did someone do something which caused an angry response in you? Sorry to say it, but that person didn't *make* you angry. They have no control over your emotions. What they said or did was completely neutral. You *chose* to react by feeling angry. I know that's hard to swallow, but it's true. Accepting your choice to feel angry in that situation is the first step to ridding yourself of those annoying negative thoughts.

We are acting like a schoolyard bully when we allow negative thoughts to enter and linger in our mind. The problem is, we are not only the bully, we're the victim. We do this when we:

- **Feel like everything is black or white**. There are no absolutes in life. Others finding fault in you or your work does not make you a failure. You made a mistake. We all do. Margarita Tartikovsky says it best, "You are not a success at 100% and a total failure at 98%."

- **Feel like it's all or nothing, always or never**. Again, no absolutes. Bad things don't *always* happen to you. Yes, you may be getting more than your fair share lately. Remember Day 1?

Count your blessings. Keep your focus on the donut, not the hole.

- **Feel like you should or shouldn't do something**. Obviously, there are some things you shouldn't legally do. But generally, you can do what you choose. Your choice may have consequences, but you always have a choice. Also, don't apply the concept of should and shouldn't to others. It's not your right to decide if others should be a certain way, or shouldn't do something.

- **Feel responsible for things outside your control**. If it rains on the day of a big event you planned, is that your fault? Of course not. If your child fails a test at school, is that your fault? No again. These situations are both out of your control. However, the reverse of this blame game is also true. If you're miserable, it's not someone else's fault. It's yours. Ouch! I found the Serenity Prayer very helpful here.

God grant me the serenity
to accept the things I cannot change;
courage to change the things I can;
and wisdom to know the difference.

Living one day at a time;
Enjoying one moment at a time;
Accepting hardships as the pathway to peace;
Taking, as He did, this sinful world
as it is, not as I would have it;
Trusting that He will make all things right
if I surrender to His Will;
That I may be reasonably happy in this life
and supremely happy with Him
Forever in the next.
Amen.

-- Reinhold Niebuhr

- **Jump to conclusions**. This is a true test of weighing the evidence. When you try to be a mind reader, *"they don't like me,"* or a fortune teller, *"I'll never feel better,"* you are jumping to conclusions. Neither of these statements is a fact. Maybe they don't like you, but until you hear them say those words, you are jumping to a conclusion based on how they treat you.

- **Filter out the good**. We're back to the donut hole again, focusing just on what's missing or what's wrong. When we only see what's bad about our situation, we are distorting the truth. We're not weighing all the evidence. Only some of it. I call people who do this on a regular basis Million Dollar People. You could give them a million dollars, and they would complain about the denomination of the bills. Last time I checked, a million dollars is a million dollars no matter what type of bills. Celebrate, don't complain.

We bully ourselves when we say, or think, any of these things. You would console a friend who said, "no one likes me," or "I'm such a failure." You would probably try to help them see the truth of the situation. You would also encourage them to examine all the evidence. Treat yourself the same way.

Process

There are more ways to bully yourself than just the six I listed. Take time to think about each of these. As the victim of your own bullying, which ones do you allow to affect you? Which ones are the hot buttons your bully knows he can push to upset you? Why do they have the power to control you that way?

Engage

Getting to know and love yourself is often a difficult task. It is also critical to living a joy-filled life.

Get Inside Your Head. Take out a sheet of blank printer paper or construction paper. Draw an outline of your head and shoulders big enough to fill the page. Don't panic. I'm not an artist either, and I did it. No one's judging the drawing except you. Add some ears and hair, but leave the face part clear and large enough to write some words.

Now, write 20 positive words to describe yourself in the space usually reserved for the eyes, nose and mouth. That's hard for most of us to do, but keep working until you can come up with 20 positive words.

Next, cover the words you wrote. Then ask 10 close friends or family members to write a word or phrase they think describes you in the empty space outside of your head outline. They can write their name if they choose. Give them different color markers if you want to make it more colorful.

You can also use social media to gather their thoughts. Make a game of it by asking everyone to describe you using only one word or phrase.

Finally, read what everyone wrote, and compare their words to yours. Were there overlaps? Were you surprised by how others saw you? Allow yourself to accept their compliments without question. And don't try to justify their comments. Examine the evidence to see why they might believe what they wrote. For example, if they said you were kind, and you can find evidence to support that, then accept the fact that you are kind. Quit focusing on the one time you acted in an unkind way.

Think Positive. One way to combat negative thoughts is to replace them with positive ones. That is done through positive affirmations or self-talk. These are statements you create which build your self-esteem and boost your mood.

First, write 10 things in your journal you often say to yourself, or about yourself, which have damaging emotional consequences. For instance, I'm fat. I'm stupid. I'm a horrible wife and mother. Take a minute to read *Who Am I* at the end of this book. It's a poem I wrote which allows me to acknowledge my positive traits while focusing on changing the things I see as negative in my life.

Now you try. Take the 10 things you listed earlier and write them as a positive. For the thought, *I'm fat*, how about, *I accept myself as I am and work daily to become healthier*. Instead of *I'm a horrible wife and mother*, try *I strive to be a loving, affectionate wife and devoted mother*. Turn *I'm stupid* into *I always do my best*. Need help? Look back at the positive words you wrote inside your head.

Be Inspired. Take time to read scripture, a devotional, or an inspirational book. Listen to uplifting music, and focus on the lyrics. Digest their meaning and how they inspire you.

Inspiration Suggestions

Indeed, the important question in terms of becoming more peaceful isn't whether you're going to have negative thoughts – you are – it's what you choose to do with the ones that you have. Richard Carlson

You are not a success at 100% and a total failure at 98%. Margarita Tartokovsky

Self-disciplined begins with the mastery of your thoughts. If you don't control what you think, you can't control what you do. Simply, self-discipline enables you to think first and act afterward. Napoleon Hill

Why do I stand up here? Anybody? I stand upon my desk to remind myself that we must constantly look at things in a different way. Robin Williams in Dead Poet's Society

Song – Speak Life by Toby Mac*

Song – Hello, My Name Is by Matthew West*

Song – Greatest Love of All by Whitney Houston*

*Video available at https://sadnesstojoy.com/inspiration/music

Reflect

1. What did you think, talk, and post about today? Were you able to stay focused on the donut (your strengths and positive traits), or did you spend the day focused on the hole (your weaknesses, mistakes, and negative traits)?

2. How will you implement what you discovered today to help you find joy?

3. How do you bully yourself with your self-talk? Write down 10 negative self-talk statements, and rephrase them from a more positive perspective.

4. Which of the Inspiration Suggestions did you choose? What stood out that you'd like to remember?

5. Go to https://sadnesstojoy.com/forum/21days, and share what you think about bullying yourself with your negative thoughts.

Day 5: Have Faith

You're still here. That's great! I'm so proud of you for getting through that rough stretch. Today on our journey we're going to sit down a bit and rest. The hardest thing we're going to do today is... think. However, I don't want us to lose ground. So while we're resting, let's contemplate the creation of the universe and our role in it. Who's really in control?

Was there a big bang, or did God create the heavens and the earth? This is one of the most controversial topics I know. Here's another. Did man evolve or was he created in God's image?

Everyone is entitled to believe what they want about how the world got here and how they were created. I fall strongly on the side of the presence of God. Some feel believing in God requires them to commit to some religion, so they refer to their higher power instead. Others call him Allah or Jehovah. Is there a common thread? There is! They all, no matter what name is used, believe a power greater than themselves created the universe and controls everything in it.

I believe that power is God. I believe he created the birds and the flowers. He controls the tides, moon, and rotation of the earth. He brings the breeze and the rain. And he controls life. All life. Including mine. I believe it's all well-planned, and things happen according to that plan.

Honestly, sometimes I think God's plan stinks. But every time I think this, I'm reminded I live in a world filled with evil. I may think I have a better plan, but I'm reminded that he is God, and I am not. He sees the whole plan from beginning to end. I only see my small part at this very moment in time. I can't possibly understand from this fractional view how everything fits together or why bad things happen. I just know I trust that no matter what happens in my life, good or bad, God's ultimate plan is for me to be in heaven with him, and I trust that plan.

God amazes me each time I watch the waves roll in and out on the beach near my home. As I watch the beautiful sunsets and the rain which provides nourishment for the plants and flowers I love. However, there was a time I wasn't amazed by God; I was angry with him. This was one of those times when I didn't care for what I thought was his plan. At all.

When I was 14, I was the victim of a violent crime. The God I trusted to protect me, hadn't. I blamed him for what evil men had done to me. But why hadn't he protected me and kept me safe? I couldn't find answers, so I walked away from God and decided I was better off on my own. I decided I had a better plan. A plan to control everything to keep myself safe.

Forty years later, in my darkest moment following a complete emotional breakdown, I decided my plan hadn't worked out all that well. So I reached out to God, because deep down, I knew only he could help me. While my faith had been shattered, it had never died.

Now, I'm almost three years on the other side of that breakdown, and without a doubt, God has helped me through. He has given me strength to face tough times, courage to face new trials, and peace every second of this journey. He's done that in several ways.

While reading my Bible, I've seen how many messed up people God used to do great things. We think of the men and women of the Bible as being these great saints. But they weren't. They were ordinary people with messed up lives just like me.

During my prayer time, I've released my problems to God. I hand them over to him multiple times a day and just say, "Here they are God. I can't fix them, but I know you can. But if you don't, I know there's a reason why."

At weekly church services, God provided friends and family to surround me and support me. He provided a message which often seemed directed straight at me, as if I was the only one listening, although several others said the same thing.

And probably the most instrumental in keeping my mind focused on God's love for me and his power over my problems was listening to inspirational music. God has always spoken to me the most clearly through music. Why don't you head back to Day 21 and sneak a peek at the Music Challenge?

Filling my heart with God's Word through music kept me from focusing on that pesky donut hole, all that was wrong and missing in my life. Instead it kept me focused on God's love for me, his desire to help me, and his power in my life.

Have you been hurt by the evil in this world? Have you been hurt by evil desires in your own life? By poor choices? He can help you too, if you'll let him. So find the way to connect that works best for you and start today.

It's time to surrender to the spirit inside which is leading you to a greater understanding of God, his role in your life, and the guidance and direction he provides if you'll just listen. Tune in to the spirit speaking within you. You have no power over your circumstances or your emotions which God has not given you. Have faith in the creator of the universe. If he can do all that, he can certainly provide for your needs and direct your path.

Process

In times of crisis, who do you call on for help? A friend? A family member? Or God?

Faith-based decisions are very personal. Not everyone believes in God, or even a higher power. They believe everything happens by chance. Is that you right now? All I ask today is to consider the possibility there is a God. That's it. I'm not asking you to make any public proclamation of faith. Just consider it.

If you are strong in your faith, lean on it in times of trouble. However, if you aren't sure about all this, I urge you to learn more. There are some great books out there on the Christian faith. I would highly recommend you read

The Case for Faith: A Journalist Investigates the Toughest Objections to Christianity,[1] or *The Case for Christ: A Journalist's Personal Investigation of the Evidence for Jesus,*[2] both by Lee Strobel.

Author's Note: Additional resources providing insight into Christianity can be found on my website at https://sadnesstojoy.com/resources/bible-study-scripture.

Engage

Take time to acknowledge God may be real. Studies can show why scientists believe things from the Bible did or didn't happen, but there is no scientific proof God does not exist.

Explore Creation. Get outside, because that's where creation happens. Go to the ocean, the forest, or whatever natural habitat is nearby. If you aren't near any of those, get away from buildings and lights, and stare at the stars. As you look at these things, consider how they got there.

Let's take the ocean. How do the waves know where to be and what to do? How do they know where to stop? Why don't they just keep rolling up the beach?

Look at the forest. Where did all those trees and plants come from? Why the variety? What causes some to grow in one area and not in others?

What about the animals? Who decided the skin of a rhinoceros should ooze a pink liquid which protects its skin from sunburn? Who created the honeycomb structure of a tortoise shell to allow it to carry it's up to 600 lb. weight?

Finally, think about the stars and planets. How did they get there? What causes some to twinkle brighter than others? Why are they in the same place night after night?

Is it even possible these things happened by chance?

In your journal, record your thoughts about whether these things happened by chance or were created by God.

Be Inspired. Take time to read scripture, a devotional, or an inspirational book. Listen to uplifting music, and focus on the lyrics. Digest their meaning and how they inspire you

Inspiration Suggestions

> *You made all the delicate, inner parts of my body and knit me together in my mother's womb. Psalm 139:13 (NLT)*
>
> *God, the Lord, created the heavens and stretched them out. He created the earth and everything in it. He gives breath to everyone, life to everyone who walks the earth. Isaiah 42:5 (NLT)*
>
> *Song – Through All of It by Colton Dixon**
>
> *Song – My Story by Big Daddy Weave**
>
> *Song – God's Not Dead by News Boys**
>
> *Song – He Is with You by Mandisa**
>
> *Song – Trust in You by Lauren Daigle**
>
> **Video available at https://sadnesstojoy.com/inspiration/music*

Reflect

1. What did you think, talk, and post about today? Were you able to stay focused on the donut (there is a God in control even when things seem out of control), or did you spend the day focused on the hole (you're on your own when circumstances are out of control)?

2. How will you implement what you discovered today to help you find joy?

3. Will the knowledge God may be real change how you deal with crisis or uncertain times in your life? Why or why not?

4. Which of the Inspiration Suggestions did you choose? What stood out that you'd like to remember?

5. Go to https://sadnesstojoy.com/forum/21days, and share your thoughts about faith and how it provides support in times of trouble.

Day 6: Get Up and Move

Wasn't yesterday a nice break to rest and rejuvenate? Were you able to get your spirit filled with hope for the remainder of our journey? I hope so. But now, break time is over. Let's get back up and get moving. Literally!

========================

Getting out of bed is too hard.

I don't want to do anything but lie here.

I don't have enough energy to do anything.

Sound familiar? These are things people who feel sad, depressed or overwhelmed might say.

The truth is, Newton had it right on this one – a body in motion stays in motion; a body at rest stays at rest. His law of motion explains how an object is impacted by the forces around it. In our case, we're more concerned about the forces inside it, our emotions, but I believe the theory still applies.

Our emotions play a large part in motivating us to stay put. When we don't feel good, we just want to lay around and be left alone. If we are physically ill, rest is probably the best thing. Quite the opposite is true with mental illness. Why's that?

Physical activity increases chemicals in the brain which can boost our mood. Even a 10- to 15-minute walk can help you feel better.[1] If you're not able to take a walk, or have access to outside spaces, turn on some music you like and dance. Come on – nobody's watching.

Lack of physical activity has the opposite effect on our mood. Scientists from the University of Maryland, found unhappy people watch 20% more television than people who proclaim to be happy.[2] I believe that holds true for computers and cell phones as well. They offer an escape. A chance to isolate yourself. They fill your time with mind-numbing games and apps to avoid facing the real world. Sneak over and check out the Electronics Challenge on Day 21. Bottom line – turn off those electronics. Instead, get up and move.

What has worked for me is using a pedometer to measure my activity. I aim for 7,000 to 10,000 steps per day. I'll be honest, when I first started I was aiming for 2,000 to 3,000 steps per day. It's about progress, not perfection.

Get yourself an inexpensive pedometer. Mine cost about $10 and clips on my waist band or shoe laces. Use it for a couple of days to determine how many steps you currently get. Average the steps and add 1,000. That's your starting goal. From there, just add 1,000 steps each time you've met your current goal for a week.

Process

How would you rate your current level of physical activity? Are there physical limitations preventing you from being more physically active? If so, are they limitations you can overcome, or will you need to think outside the box when planning physical activity? Just a hint, weight CAN be overcome? Yes it takes time and effort, but it can be overcome? Disease and disability are things which would require outside-the-box thinking. Here are a few fitness sites offering ideas for everything from a seated chair workout for those with limited mobility to a full-blown boot camp. You can also find goal-setting advice and fitness tracking apps.

- Mayo Clinic - http://mayocl.in/1W4oV4M

- Spark People - http://bit.ly/2dSzQPo

- Fitness Magazine - http://bit.ly/2eaSgcE

- Map My Fitness - http://bit.ly/1DnTfdG

What's holding you back?

Engage

Getting started is the hardest part. Some people find it easier to jump right in, while others need a little more time to adjust to the idea.

Plan and Track Your Movement. Use a calendar, or the blank Physical Activity Plan provided, to set some goals for yourself. Then plan a week's worth of activity. Start simple. Your first goal may be to get out of bed at the same time every morning, get cleaned up, dressed, and have breakfast. If that's improvement for you, it's perfect. Start there.

Others may already be leading a relatively normal lifestyle and just need to add a little movement. That's great. Plan to add 15-30 minutes per day of walking, gardening, dancing, or aerobic activity.

The point is to set goals and track your progress. Use the Physical Activity Tracker provided to do that. Remember, it's about progress, not perfection. Add a little bit more each week or so to keep yourself challenged.

Be Inspired. Take time to read scripture, a devotional, or an inspirational book. Listen to uplifting music, and focus on the lyrics. Digest their meaning and how they inspire you.

Inspiration Suggestions

Just do it. ™ *Nike*

Take care of your body. It's the only place you have to live. Jim Rohn

The reason I exercise is for the quality of life I enjoy. Kenneth H. Cooper

The secret of getting ahead is getting started. Mark Twain

> *Strive for progress, not perfection. Unknown*

Reflect

1. What did you think, talk, and post about today? Were you able to stay focused on the donut (you can feel better just by being more active), or did you spend the day focused on the hole (nothing will make you feel better so why try)?

2. How will you implement what you discovered today to help you find joy?

3. How do you currently stay active and healthy?

4. What goals have you set for yourself? Are they comfortable or challenging?

5. What obstacles will you need to overcome to be more physically active? How will you overcome them?

6. Which of the Inspiration Suggestions did you choose? What stood out that you'd like to remember?

7. Go to https://sadnesstojoy.com/forum/21days, and share your thoughts about adding more physical activity to your life.

Day 7: Practice Enjoying Life

Nobody enjoys exercise. Okay some people do, but I'm not one of them. I enjoy being physically active though. Hopefully you got yourself up moving around yesterday. It may have been the first time in a while. That's great! It may not have been great fun, but hopefully you got a little enjoyment out of it.

Speaking of getting enjoyment, we've been doing a lot of hard work on our journey thus far. I think today we will take a little time to stop and enjoy it. I think I see a playground off to the right. Come on; let's have some fun.

I used to enjoy going to theme parks, on picnics, and playing games with friends and family. I just don't enjoy those things anymore.

I don't even want to go hang out with friends anymore. It brings me down. I've gained 20 pounds, have wrinkles everywhere, and hair color doesn't even cover the gray. I don't feel pretty anymore.

Have you said something similar recently yourself? Have you found you don't enjoy doing things you used to enjoy?

Everyone has a teenage girl or boy inside them worrying about what others will think. I like what Dr. Seuss says on the subject, "Be who you are and say what you feel, because those who mind don't matter and those who matter don't mind." So quit worrying about what others think. Just enjoy where you are and what you're doing. I'm not saying don't make changes to improve if there's something you don't like, but enjoy life in the process of changing.

Is there a reason you don't enjoy certain activities anymore? If not, it's time to start doing them again – whether you feel like it or not. Don't let your emotions drive your day! You may need to start going places and doing things which currently make you feel uncomfortable. But the more you do them, the easier they will get.

If the things you used to do are associated with bad memories, try something new. Start small. Why not surprise your spouse, significant other, child or friend for lunch one day? Spend a day enjoying the cultural arts at a museum or local festival. Enjoy nature by taking a bike ride, or walk through a local park. Take the scenic route for once. Or go completely crazy, put on some music from a happy time and dance, get some paints, create something, or go pile up some leaves or snow and take a flying leap into it.

Process

Living a life you don't enjoy is entirely within your control to change. It takes effort, but you can learn to enjoy life again. Start by changing one thing. Then add others as you feel comfortable. Think about some things you used to do but don't anymore. Really think about it. What makes you happy? What do you enjoy doing?

Engage

The first step in learning to enjoy life is to admit you don't enjoy what you have right now. But that acknowledgment comes with a commitment that nothing you currently do is safe from the cutting table. To make room for new enjoyable habits, unhealthy ones will need to go.

Things I Enjoy. In your journal, list 10 things you would enjoy doing. Don't worry about who would do it with you, ability level, or what others might think, just list them. For instance, my list would include dancing, ice skating, karaoke – none of which I have any ability in. Nevertheless, I enjoy doing them.

Now pick one from your list, and make it happen. Schedule time this week to either do it or start the planning process.

Next list 10 things you do well. Your strengths. The things you feel confident about and make you feel good emotionally. For instance, my list would include organizing things, planning events, and teaching Bible study. These are all things I believe I do well and enjoy doing.

Now pick one from this list, and make it happen. Schedule time this week to either do it or start the planning process.

Happy Holidays. People struggling with their emotions often have a difficult time around the holidays. Everybody else is happy and wants to have fun, while you play the part of Scrooge or Grinch this holiday season. However, the holidays are a lonely time for many people. You are not alone. While being good to yourself won't erase feelings of loneliness at the holidays, taking special care of yourself can help you feel better.

In your journal, list 10 things you enjoy, or used to enjoy, about the holidays. If something has taken the joy from these activities, do something different. Take each item on the list, and plan how you can make it enjoyable again. If an item is too painful to continue, plan a way to replace it. Include things which make you feel good. Get a massage, buy a new outfit, take a trip, or throw a party. If it feels good, give yourself permission to do it.

Also, helping others gets your mind off yourself. The holidays present multiple opportunities to do that. Adopt a family, volunteer at a shelter, go caroling at an assisted living facility or wrap presents for a busy mom.

Be Inspired. Take time to read scripture, a devotional, or an inspirational book. Listen to uplifting music, and focus on the lyrics. Digest their meaning and how they inspire you.

Inspiration Suggestions

Be who you are and say what you feel, because those who mind don't matter and those who matter don't mind. Dr. Seuss

Why should we worry about what others think of us, do we have more confidence in their opinions than we do of our own? Brigham Young

And I'll sit back and say to myself, "My friend, you have enough stored away for years to come. Now take it easy! Eat, drink, and be merry!" Luke 12:19 (NLT)

Song – Free to be Me by Francesca Battistelli*

Song – Thrive by Casting Crowns*

Song – Good to Be Alive by Jason Gray*

*Video available at https://sadnesstojoy.com/inspiration/music

Reflect

1. What did you think, talk, and post about today? Were you able to stay focused on the donut (living a life you enjoy is within your control), or did you spend the day focused on the hole (your life is miserable and there's nothing you can do to change it)?

2. How will you implement what you discovered today to help you find joy?

3. What area of your life do you feel negatively affects your emotions? Why?

4. What could you do to start enjoying that aspect of your life more?

5. What obstacles will you need to overcome to begin enjoying it? How will you overcome them?

6. Did you have a hard time listing 10 things you would enjoy and 10 things you feel you do well? Why do you think that is?

7. Which of the Inspiration Suggestions did you choose? What stood out that you'd like to remember?

8. Go to https://sadnesstojoy.com/forum/21days, and share your thoughts about learning to enjoy life.

Day 8: Master Your Mind and Habits

Can you believe it? We are a third of the way through our journey. It hasn't been that bad, has it? After all, we've taken time to rest and play along the way. Hopefully you're starting to develop some new habits.

I've saved this day until now for a reason. There's some rough terrain ahead. You've gotten a chance to warm-up, and now it's time for the real workout. Just like on Day 4, the best way to get through it is to take my hand and step exactly in my footsteps. Remember, I've already navigated through this before. I know the easiest route. I got through it. You can too. Take a deep breath, hold on tight, and let's do it together.

My therapist used to tell me, "keep your head where your feet are planted." She wanted me to forget what happened yesterday, and quit thinking about what might happen tomorrow. She'd say, "You aren't in those places. You're right here, right now. Focus on that."

She also repeatedly reminded me obsessing over the past brings on depression. Obsessing over the future, anxiety. I quickly discovered I was blessed with both. It's difficult to be focused on the current moment when your brain is working on 12 other problems or emotions at the same time.

Then I realized she was right. If things were going to change, I needed to focus my energy on one thing at a time. I had to keep my head where my feet were planted, right then and there, and being constantly aware of my extraneous thoughts and emotions was the only way to manage them.

Over time, I learned to toss aside anything unrelated to what was happening right that minute. However, self-awareness didn't happen overnight, and it can't be learned in a book. It can only be achieved through self-reflection.[1]

We talked about self-awareness on Day 2 – How Food Affects Your Mood and again on Day 6 – Get Up and Move. In both cases, we used a tracking method to monitor progress toward a positive change in our behavior. Those tracking methods were very specific to the task at hand.

However, the following four-step self-awareness process can be used with any change you want to make: Plan, Implement, Reflect, and Adjust (PIRA). Here's how it works.

- **PLAN** – set goals, and map out steps to achieve them. Use the daily activities we've discussed. For instance, you could eat healthier, add more physical activity, or carve out time to build your faith. Be sure to list obstacles which may interfere, and then plan strategies to overcome them.

- **IMPLEMENT** – carry out your plan step-by-step. If obstacles come up, use the strategies you developed in your plan. If an unplanned obstacle comes up, pause to think before you respond.

- **REFLECT** – at the end of each goal period (day/week/month), reflect on your plan. Did it go the way you hoped? If not, why? Did it go better than you hoped? Great! Why do you think that was the case?

- **ADJUST** – change whatever didn't go the way you hoped. The unexpected obstacle, for instance. Plan how you will overcome it next time.

Using the **PIRA** process helps with self-awareness by keeping your mind focused on one activity at a time. Ask yourself how what you're doing moves you closer to your goal? If it doesn't, how can you change what you're doing so it does align with your goal? If today's plan didn't go the way you hoped, reflect and adjust your plan for tomorrow. This allows you to start each day with renewed hope. These small daily adjustments will make the difference. We'll practice this in the *Engage* section by establishing two daily goals.

Without goals, your life lacks meaning and purpose. You'll wander aimlessly through your life never seeming to find time to make things better. You'll end up surviving rather than thriving. Your goals should focus on what you value and hope to accomplish long-term. The goal of this book is to help you achieve a joy-filled life, so let your goals reflect that.

Process

Learning to be more aware of your thoughts and emotions takes time and practice. Simplifying your life, which we'll talk about on Day 13, will help. By lessening your obligations, you'll free up your mind to focus on things that matter.

For instance, what activities are you doing right now only to make someone else happy? It's time to gracefully bow out. Just let them know you'll be stepping back for a while to focus on other obligations.

Remember the 12 other problems and emotions I mentioned your brain was distracted by earlier? Figure out how to let them go, because the less you do, the less you have to worry about. And spending less time worrying will free your brain up to better manage your current actions, thoughts, and emotions.

So think about it for a minute. What actions, thoughts or emotions are keeping you from a joy-filled life? Which one, if changed, would have the greatest impact? Let's start there.

Engage

Practicing the **PIRA** process takes time. And it won't be comfortable at first. In fact, it will feel like extra work for no reason. However, once you start, you'll realize it saves you time, gets you closer to achieving positive change in your life, and is well worth the effort.

PIRA Goal Tracker. In addition to the **PIRA** Goal Sheet provided, you'll also need a weekly calendar. While a monthly calendar allows you to see all the goals on one page, at the daily goal level, you'll probably need more space to write than it gives.

Follow the **PIRA** process to plan one or two monthly goals. Then break those down to create weekly goals and a little further still to create daily goals. At the daily level, you'll need to decide what time to work on your goals. In other words, make a specific appointment with yourself. Then keep it.

Why don't we walk through the process together? You may have discovered on Day 4 that disputing negative thoughts was a real challenge for you. As a result, you want to focus on changing that behavior. Your monthly goal will be to evict the bully inside your head. So start by writing that goal at the end of the month. Now you need to figure out how you will accomplish it?

Week one needs to be spent completing the *Get Inside Your Head* activity. You might break that down into two days. One to come up with your words and a second to solicit words from friends and family. Thirty minutes to an hour each day should suffice. You can use social media as a time saver. Create a post explaining your assignment, and ask them to list one word or phrase they believe describes you. The remainder of the week could be spent reflecting on the words, examining the evidence, and deciding what it would take to believe it. Fifteen minutes a day for reflection should be fine.

Week two you could spend a day or two developing positive self-talk. Fifteen to thirty minutes each should do it. The remainder of the week could be spent creating resources to help you remember them. For instance, you could create some flip cards to carry with you, a poster for the fridge, or Post-it notes to place around the house. Be creative. Plan one day to shop for supplies, then one or more for the creative process. You could spend 30 minutes to several hours on this depending on your level of creativity. I could spend several hours creating what my daughter-in-law would spend 30 minutes doing, and it wouldn't be even remotely as good. But it's mine. Don't judge yourself. Just have fun with it.

Week three and four could be spent practicing and monitoring your progress. Spend a day creating a *Did I...* chart? Spend 30 minutes to an hour on this. Start with the negative thoughts I listed on Day 4, and then add your own. For instance, did I feel like everything was black and white today? Did I jump to conclusions today? Spend about 15 to 30 minutes each day thereafter reflecting on the chart. If the answer to any of the questions is yes, use the reflection and adjustment process to set yourself up to avoid those thoughts the following day. This is where the change will happen; where you will meet your goal of evicting the bully.

At the end of the month, do a final reflection. Review where you were at the beginning of the month. Assess how well you met your daily and weekly goals. Did you evict that bully? If not, is he at least on notice his days are numbered? You may not have met your goal, but that's okay. I guarantee if you've been putting in the effort, you are closer than you were when you started. Use the **PIRA** process to decide how you need to adjust as you continue to dispute your negative thoughts. Then just keep refining the process until you achieve your goal.

Pick Two. Your bigger monthly goals may be about changing habits, saving money, losing weight, refinishing the bathroom, etc. In addition to those goals which are broken down to the daily level, set two additional daily goals. These will be small goals unrelated to your monthly goals.

For instance, I have a repeating daily goal to get 10,000 steps in per day. If I say I need to exercise more but only monitor once a week or once a month, too much time has passed to be effective. I need to hold myself accountable daily.

Another example would be setting an additional daily goal to be up by five am to go to the gym before work. Why is it important for me to plan that in advance? It will require an early bedtime, advance preparation of a gym bag with clothes picked out, etc. I can assure you the gym will not happen if I don't plan it in advance.

I prefer to plan the next day's goals at night. You may prefer to do it first thing in the morning. Either way is fine.

Record your two daily goals in your journal, and schedule time on your calendar to complete them.

Be Inspired. Take time to read scripture, a devotional, or an inspirational book. Listen to uplifting music, and focus on the lyrics. Digest their meaning and how they inspire you.

Inspiration Suggestions

The ability to be in the present moment is a major component of mental wellness. Abraham Maslow

Carpe diem. Seize the day, boys. Make your lives extraordinary. Robin Williams in Dead Poets Society

When it is obvious that the goals cannot be reached, don't adjust the goals, adjust the action steps. Confucius

Setting a goal is not the main thing. It is deciding how you will go about achieving it, and staying with that plan. Tom Landry

Don't copy the behavior and customs of this world, but let God transform you into a new person by changing the way you think. Then you will learn to know God's will for you, which is good and pleasing and perfect. Romans 12:2 (NLT)

Reflect

1. What did you think, talk, and post about today? Were you able to stay focused on the donut (tomorrow can be better than today if you will just think about what didn't go well today and make small changes when you try again tomorrow), or did you spend the day focused on the hole (things will never change, you don't have the willpower or discipline to change, it's just too hard)?

2. How will you implement what you discovered today to help you find joy?

3. How does it make you feel to think about setting goals? Why do you think you feel that way?

4. What obstacles will you need to overcome to use the **PIRA** process? How will you overcome them?

5. What did you set for your first monthly goal? Did you have trouble breaking it down into smaller steps? Remember, it does get easier, so don't give up.

6. How did you do with your daily goals? What can you do differently to help you be more successful?

7. Which of the Inspiration Suggestions did you choose? What stood out that you'd like to remember?

8. Go to https://sadnesstojoy.com/forum/21days, and share your thoughts about self-awareness and tracking your progress toward positive habit changes.

Day 9: Remember Happy Times

You made it through that challenging part of our journey and came back for another day. You must be strong and determined, because goal setting and planning are difficult and time-consuming. Great job!

It's time now for another break from all our hard work. I think we need to spend a little more time focusing on enjoying life. What has been your favorite part of the journey so far? I'm sure it's probably different than mine, but that's okay. We each enjoy different things.

Looking back at things we've enjoyed helps make the hard parts of the journey a little easier. The same applies to our life. Despite what you may be thinking right now, life has not always been this rough. You have had some happy times along the way. You may have to look hard to find them, but they are there. I promise. Let's take a trip down memory lane today and re-live some of those happy times.

As a cheerleader, the most memorable moment each year was that first football game of the season. The sun was bright as the crowd stood cheering on their team. And the fall breeze blew excitement through the air. I still remember those moments as if they were yesterday.

Later, as a new mom, I remember the nurse saying, "Push. Breathe. *Ha-he-he-hoo.*" Then she said, "Again! It won't be long now." Finally, he appeared. Through the tears, I could see the beautiful eyes, gorgeous red hair, and cute little pucker. My heart overflowed with love when I held him. There's nothing like the birth of your first child. Even though things went terribly wrong for me after the birth, almost costing me my life, I still remember those moments with great joy.

Do you remember those *firsts?* What are those moments in your life? The ones you will always remember? The ones which fill your heart with joy just thinking about them. Has it been awhile since you had one of those moments? Do you seem to have more unhappy times than happy lately?

Fortunately, the nice thing about those happy moments is, they're always there. They are only a thought away. That's why I take pictures of everything. When I'm down in the dumps, I can pull out those pictures and re-live those happy memories. My family just needs to say the word Monopoly and I break out in a smile.

It's time to start remembering those happy times and re-living them. Why not create a memory book, a photo album, or write the story of your life using ONLY the happy times? Take time today to talk with a friend or family member and recount your happy memories.

Some people discount this as living in the past. I see their point, because if all you can do is relive the glory days, they're right. That's not healthy. However, as long as you are continuing to make new ones, using those old memories to remind you of the good times you've had is perfectly healthy.

It's also important to start each day with a positive outlook. Each morning when the sun rises, you have a fresh start. No baggage from yesterday allowed. Pack it up, and leave it there, because anything is possible today.

Start by believing the best about what might happen today. My daughter and I used to sing a song in the morning. It is one of those happy memories I cherish. It's based on Psalm 118:24 - This is the day that the LORD has made; let us rejoice and be glad in it.

Process

When my father passed away, I made something called a memory card. I created a postcard size sheet with one line on it – *My favorite memory of Jimmy is....* That's it. We handed these cards out at the visitation and funeral.

Then, my daughter collected the completed ones in a basket. Over the next few days, those memories from childhood friends, coworkers, and distant relatives gave us a new understanding of my dad. We saw him through a fresh set of eyes. Those memory cards still bring me joy today.

What happy times do you remember? How does it make you feel when you recall them? Don't wait until someone is gone to discover all the interesting things about them. Ask now. Share your stories, and listen to theirs. It will bring a smile to your face and maybe, just maybe, a good mood-boosting belly laugh will well up and fall out.

Engage

Enjoying the happy memories from your past must be balanced with recognition of the happy things around you today. You also need to be able to dream of happy times in your future.

I Like Myself. In your journal, list 10-15 things you like about yourself. For instance, my list would include my friendliness, smile, good health, and petite feet. You notice my waistline is nowhere on that list. Don't forget to ask all the people who care about you what they like about you.

Whenever you find something you don't like about yourself, pull out this list. Let it remind you of all you do like. There's that donut again. Focus on what you like, not what you don't like.

Oh yeah, about that waistline. It is on the don't like list right now, but it doesn't have to stay that way. Create a list of three things you don't like about yourself. Only three. Now pick one from this list, and use the **PIRA** process to plan how you will convert it over to the *Like* list.

Three Good Things. Every morning before lunch, write down one good thing that happened that morning. Don't eat your lunch until you come up with at least one good thing. Then think about what made it good.

Repeat this process again after work or school and again before bed. At the end of each day, you will have listed three things that went well that day.

This helps keep you focused on what's going right rather than what's going wrong.

Be Inspired. Take time to read scripture, a devotional, or an inspirational book. Listen to uplifting music, and focus on the lyrics. Digest their meaning and how they inspire you.

Inspiration Suggestions

Most folks are about as happy as they make up their minds to be. Abraham Lincoln

Being happy doesn't mean that everything is perfect. It means that you've decided to look beyond the imperfections. Gerard Way

A cheerful heart does good like medicine, but a broken spirit makes one sick. Proverbs 17:22 (TLB)

Song – Happy by Pharrell Williams*

Song – Don't Worry be Happy by Bobby McFerrin*

*Video available at https://sadnesstojoy.com/inspiration/music

Reflect

1. What did you think, talk, and post about today? Were you able to stay focused on the donut (all the happy times you've had), or did you spend the day focused on the hole (all the unhappy things that have happened throughout your life or are happening right now)?

2. How will you implement what you discovered today to help you find joy?

3. What does happiness mean to you? What would it look like in your life?

4. Think about three happy memories from your childhood or earlier adult life. What makes them memorable? Why did they make you happy? Could you re-create them?

5. What can you do today to start recording your happy memories to look back on later?

6. Which of the Inspiration Suggestions did you choose? What stood out that you'd like to remember?

7. Go to https://sadnesstojoy.com/forum/21days, and share your thoughts about remembering the happy times from your past.

Day 10: Practice Prayer and Meditation

Are you feeling a little better after spending time in those happy memories? Chances are you had forgotten a few until you forced yourself to think about them. I hope your memories gave you as much joy as mine did.

Now, let's not forget to go back and count those as blessings. While we're at it, let's step away from our journey for another opportunity to rest our body and our spirit. Let's take some time to thank God for the happy times and ask for his help and guidance for the remainder of our journey.

Now I lay me down to sleep...

God is great, God is good...

These were some of the early prayers I learned as a child. They were simple and rhythmic to make it easy for children to learn and remember.

Praying is simply asking God to fulfill your need or to offer thanks for his blessings. Prayers can be simple or elaborate but should be heartfelt. The rote prayers above are okay as a child, because we may not yet understand the power of God in meeting the needs of his children. However, as an adult, prayers should be more a conversation than a recitation.

Why don't people pray? Some say they feel silly talking to the air. I've also heard it's because they don't need anything right now. They'll pray when they need something. Let's examine that last one a little more closely.

Let's say your parents live in another city. You never seem to get time to call them except when you need something. How do you think they will respond? I suspect they will be hurt. They may give you what you need; however, the fact you only want to talk when they can give you something must really sting. Just like our parents, God wants to be in a relationship with you. He doesn't just want to be your genie in a bottle called out when you need something.

Another excuse is, "it's the pastor's job to pray for the people. Not mine." However, Galatians 6:2 says, "Bear one another's burdens, and so fulfill the law of Christ." Does that sound like it is only the pastor's job to pray for the people? Not to me. 1 Thessalonians 5:11 says it another way, "So encourage each other and build each other up, just as you are already doing." I think it's clear God expects us to care for the physical and spiritual needs of others.

Process

When we read a scripture, devotional, or inspiring quote we tend to think about it for a while. That is called meditating. Meditation is an extension of prayer. The quiet time you spend thinking about what you read or requested is an opportunity for God to speak back to you. It's a chance to ask God what he wants you to do with your prayer requests or the scripture you read.

Meditation doesn't require you to make funny noises or sit in peculiar positions like you've seen on TV. Just sit in a quiet place and let your mind focus on what you read or requested. What do prayer and meditation look like in your life? If they don't currently exist, what's holding you back?

Engage

Prayer is a conversation between you and God. Plan that time wisely.

Create a Prayer Journal. Get yourself a pretty journal, a simple 3-ring binder, or use the Prayer Journal page provided. Start a fresh page each day.

Record the date, then start recording the people you know who need prayer. It could be a friend, family member, or coworker. Someone you need to forgive for hurting you. It could even be someone, or some group of people, half way around the world struggling in a war or natural disaster. Leave space by each request to record the date it is answered and the outcome.

Now start writing prayer requests for yourself. Be specific. For instance, "I need to find $50 more in my budget to pay the bills this month." Or, "I need the courage to ask for a flexible schedule to get my kids to and from school, a 2% raise, or a one-week extension on my current project." Again, leave space for answered prayers.

Follow the same process each day, but don't repeat anything from a previous day. New things can be big or small requests. It may be as simple as, "God, help me." Or as specific as, "my spouse passed away overnight. Give me strength to get out of bed and face a day without him. Give compassion to the funeral home staff as they assist me today. Bring friends to support and provide for me today since I'm unable to do it for myself."

Now, start praying over this list every morning and evening. Yes, it's okay to leave your eyes open when you pray. It's also okay to read from a list, flipping back to previous days so you can remember ongoing prayer needs. If you can't find time twice a day, start with once a day. Just start.

As you begin to see prayers answered, and you will, record the date and outcome of each answered prayer. Then highlight through that request so you can stop praying about it. Now add it to your prayer list for today as a Praise. Don't forget to include other praises such as a new job or a new baby.

Be Inspired. Take time to read scripture, a devotional, or an inspirational book. Listen to uplifting music, and focus on the lyrics. Digest their meaning and how they inspire you.

Inspiration Suggestions

One day Jesus told his disciples a story to show that they should always pray and never give up. Luke 18:1 (NLT)

Don't worry about anything; instead, pray about everything. Tell God what you need, and thank him for all he has done. Then you will experience God's peace, which exceeds anything we can understand. His peace will guard your hearts and minds as you live in Christ Jesus. Philippians 4:6-7 (NLT)

Song – Cast My Cares by Finding Favour*

Song – Just Be Held by Casting Crowns*

Song – Cry Out to Jesus by Third Day*

*Video available at https://sadnesstojoy.com/inspiration/music

Reflect

1. What did you think, talk, and post about today? Were you able to stay focused on the donut (the knowledge you're not alone, you have a God waiting to talk to you and help you), or did you spend the day focused on the hole (the misconception that you're alone, so no one hears you or cares)?

2. How will you implement what you discovered today to help you find joy?

3. Was writing down your prayer needs easy or difficult? Was it easier to find prayer needs for yourself or for others? Why do you think that was?

4. Did writing down the prayer needs of others give you a new perspective on your own needs? How so?

5. Have you ever prayed or meditated before? If not, why?

6. What obstacles might you need to overcome to make prayer and meditation a daily habit? How will you overcome them?

7. Which of the Inspiration Suggestions did you choose? What stood out that you'd like to remember?

8. Go to https://sadnesstojoy.com/forum/21days, and share your thoughts about prayer and meditation.

Day 11: Create Wellness Habits

Now that we know God is waiting to help us, let's ask. Since our journey brings us to a first-aid station today, we can ask for help to get better.

The first-aid station is where you go when you're sick so the doctor can prescribe something to help you get better. Since we're already here, let's pick up a prescription for some tools which will help us get better.

Being well prepared with the proper tools is the best way to complete a task. No carpenter would leave the house without his toolbelt and toolbox. Why? Because they hold everything he needs to complete the job. They're also very organized. Everything he uses regularly is on the toolbelt, and the specialty tools used less often are in the toolbox.

In our case, the task is finding joy. This requires a tool to identify and remove unhealthy habits which don't lead to joy. But we will also need tools to help us practice healthy habits which may lead to joy.

Let's look at what tools should be in our new Wellness Toolkit.

Wellness Action Plan. This is where you will use the **PIRA** process to write wellness goals, think of potential obstacles, and plan to overcome them. You will also write which tools you plan to use. Here are some examples:

- **Creative Avoidance** – purposely planning an activity to avoid a stressor or trigger (stressors make you worried or anxious, while triggers cause you to do something)

- **Healthy Diet & Exercise** – eating healthy foods, drinking plenty of water, and getting regular exercise as a support to wellness

- **Identify Triggers** – recognition of people, places, things, and events which cause you to be anxious or depressed

- **Laughter** – finding things to make you smile and laugh, such as a joke book, silly videos (YouTube has tons), or a funny movie

- **New View** – looking at your situation from a new perspective or seeing it from another person's perspective

- **Overcoming Obstacles** – identifying obstacles to wellness habit changes and planning ways to overcome them

- **Positive Self-Talk** – speaking and thinking positive things about yourself rather than negative

- **Re-Direction** – distracting yourself from an unexpected stressor or trigger, such as walking away or changing the subject

- **Relaxation Techniques** – music, meditation, soft lighting, hot bath, or massage to reduce stress and anxiety

- **Serenity Prayer** – changing what you can control (yourself) and accepting what you can't control (everything else)

- **Stop, Drop, and Rephrase** – Stop any negative thought, drop any anxiety or emotion it caused, and rephrase it more positively

- **Support Person/Group** – a compassionate, trustworthy person or group you turn to when in need

- **Symptoms Checker** – a place to chart daily symptoms of depression or anxiety

- **Worry Willow Tree** – recognition of something worrisome and a decision tree which determines your next action (see example in the journal)

Process

Everyone is in a different place on this journey. Some are starting from step one, while others are already a thousand steps in. Where you stand on this journey will determine what tools will be most beneficial for you.

Review the list, and remove any tools you won't need. These are things you've already mastered. They aren't a problem for you. For instance, you may be relatively stable and just want to add more joy to your life. If that's the case, you probably won't need the Symptoms Checker.

Now take a second look. Pick out a few you need more immediately. These will be on your toolbelt ready to grab in an instant. The remaining items will be in your toolbox, ready for those special things that come up. Prioritize the items you selected for your Toolbelt. Which three do you need the most and why? These will be the first three you work to develop.

Engage

It's time to assemble your own personal Wellness Toolkit.

Wellness Progress Report. Lasting change happens by monitoring your habits regularly and making small changes over time. Complete the Wellness Progress Report in your journal on a daily basis. It lists the habits which support a joy-filled life. Each night, review the Progress Report, and place a check mark in the box beside each habit you successfully completed that day. You may wish to copy the page first so that you will be able to use it repeatedly as you travel this journey.

Create a Wellness Toolkit (aka Wellness Action Plan). Let's start by identifying your wellness goals. Complete the Wellness Goal Sheet in your journal.

Next, overcoming obstacles often involves using one of your tools, so review the Tool Guide in your journal. It outlines the tool to use for the stressor, trigger, or obstacle you face.

Finally, use the Support Team Sheet in your journal to identify members of your support team should you need them. At the very least, your spouse, significant other, or best friend should be on your team.

Be Inspired. Take time to read scripture, a devotional, or an inspirational book. Listen to uplifting music, and focus on the lyrics. Digest their meaning and how they inspire you.

Inspiration Suggestions

You yourself, as much as anybody in the entire universe, deserve your love and attention. Buddha

To me, good health is more than just exercise and diet. It's really a point of view and a mental attitude you have about yourself. Albert Schweitzer

Planning is bringing the future into the present so that you can do something about it now. Alan Lakein

The more time you spend contemplating what you should have done... you lose valuable time planning what you can and will do. Lil Wayne

Reflect

1. What did you think, talk, and post about today? Were you able to stay focused on the donut (there are tools you can use and habits you can develop which will make you feel better), or did you spend the day focused on the hole (you've tried everything and nothing works)?

2. How will you implement what you discovered today to help you find joy?

3. What items did you take out of your toolkit? Why?

4. What items did you move to your toolbelt for immediate access? Why?

5. How does it feel to know you are learning to use the tools you need to start enjoying your life more?

6. What were your thoughts as you developed your Wellness Action Plan?

7. What obstacles might you face in using some of these tools? How will you overcome them?

8. Which of the Inspiration Suggestions did you choose? What stood out that you'd like to remember?

9. Go to https://sadnesstojoy.com/forum/21days, and share your thoughts about preparing a Wellness Action Plan.

Day 12: Identify Your Triggers

Today we've got some tricky terrain to maneuver. It's a good thing we packed so many tools. We'll need them to help us finish this journey stronger than we started. Any time you need to stop and pull out a tool, just say so. We're not in any hurry. Let's pull one of them out right now and use it to practice identifying our triggers.

Fires don't just ignite, guns don't fire by themselves, and bombs don't usually explode without help. They all have one thing in common – something triggers them.

Your emotions are the same way. Anxiety, worry, anger, grief, embarrassment and sadness. All these emotions start with a trigger. The trick to controlling these emotions is to identify the trigger.

When we have an emotional reaction to something and scream, "he made me so mad," we must first understand he didn't do anything to us. He did something, and we became angry. It follows that if we are responsible for starting the anger response, we're also responsible for stopping it. However, it's not as simple as just turning it back off.

Accepting responsibility for your emotional responses is not easy. But once you do that, you can reflect on what happened that might have caused your emotional reaction.

That means figuring out what about his action caused you to feel angry. Was it what he did or something he said? Was it the surroundings or the other people present? Maybe a combination of these? Play detective with your emotions. Replay the video in your mind. Find the clues you need to solve the mystery of your exploding emotions.

Once you finally identify a suspect, it's time to develop strategies to avoid the same emotional explosion in the future. This usually requires the use of one of the tools discussed on Day 11. Look in your Wellness Toolkit, and decide which is the best tool for the task at hand.

Your plan will need to include the following:

- Trigger or stressor

- Warning signs an emotional explosion is imminent

- Precautions to avoid an explosion (tools)

- Celebration when the threat is diffused

One way to avoid stress or worry is to do a risk assessment each time these emotions start. Ask yourself the following:

- Why is this thought or activity causing an emotional reaction? How would I rank my emotions on a scale of 1-10?

- What is it I'm afraid is going to happen? What facts are there to support this outcome? What facts are there to support a different outcome?

- How would I rank the likelihood of the anticipated outcome occurring on a scale of 1-10?

- What will I do with this new information?

Answers to these questions will provide the information you need to either release the worry due to the unlikeliness of it happening or prepare for it due to the probability of it happening. Remember to make fact-based decisions and not emotion-based ones.

Process

We all have stressors and triggers in our life which cause emotional reactions. The decision to be made is whether it will be a tremor or a full-blown earthquake. What are some things which cause you to react emotionally?

Engage

Learning to identify your triggers, and control the emotional explosions which follow, takes time and practice. Let's look at some that are giving you trouble.

Identify Your Triggers. In your journal, begin to explore what people, places, things, and events trigger your emotional explosions. Start by addressing your most recent one.

Be Inspired. Take time to read scripture, a devotional, or an inspirational book. Listen to uplifting music, and focus on the lyrics. Digest their meaning and how they inspire you.

Inspiration Suggestions

Anger begins as an inner twinge. We sense something long before it blossoms (explodes?) into an emotional tirade. If we listen to this twinge -- and follow its advice -- the emotional outburst (or in burst) is not needed. Peter McWilliams (emphasis mine)

Every day we have plenty of opportunities to get angry, stressed or offended. But what you're doing when you indulge these negative emotions is giving something outside yourself power over your happiness. You can choose to not let little things upset you. Joel Osteen

> *There is a reason for everything. Before I react with emotion, I step back and ask why, and the answer will be given to me. Unknown*
>
> *God is our refuge and strength, always ready to help in times of trouble. So, we will not fear when earthquakes come and the mountains crumble into the sea. Psalm 46:1-2 (NLT)*

Reflect

1. What did you think, talk, and post about today? Were you able to stay focused on the donut (you can control your emotional explosions), or did you spend the day focused on the hole (some people just know how to push your buttons, you can't help it)?

2. How will you implement what you discovered today to help you find joy?

3. Was it easy to identify some of your triggers or did you have a hard time?

4. What tools did you decide to use? Why?

5. Which of the Inspiration Suggestions did you choose? What stood out that you'd like to remember?

6. Go to https://sadnesstojoy.com/forum/21days, and share your thoughts about identifying your triggers and learning to defuse them.

Day 13: Learn About Depression

How well did you manage the minefield of emotional explosions yesterday? I told you it was going to be tricky. Today will be a little easier though. We're going to spend some time learning how to make the remainder of our journey a little easier.

———————————

My mind is moving so quickly; I just can't keep up.

I have so much to do; I'm not even sure where to start.

I'm so nervous I'll make a mistake.

I just can't focus, or sleep, or... I give up! I can't do this anymore!

There are several names for these types of feelings, but let's start with this – NORMAL. Everyone feels this way at one time or another. You may call it stress. Others call it anxiety. I've learned to call it unhealthy.

Work/Life Balance is a key buzz word these days. It means finding time to have a job and a personal life at the same time. The person described above is out of balance. Too much to do with no time for relaxation isn't healthy.

There are countless number of books, websites and apps to help you manage your time. Using a schedule, blocking your time, or delegating tasks, to name a few strategies they discuss. That's all well and good. However, if you have too many commitments, no amount of scheduling, blocking or delegating is going to help.

It's time to simplify. To prioritize what matters and politely step back from everything else. If that means your children only participate in one after school activity at a time, so be it. We did it, and my children turned out just fine.

The best thing you can do is to learn about boundaries. Set them, and enforce them, because people won't respect your time if you don't. An excellent resource for this is a book entitled, *Boundaries: When to Say Yes, When to Say No, to Take Control of Your Life* by Dr. Henry Cloud and Dr. John Townsend.[1] Another is *The Best Yes* by Lysa TerKeurst.[2]

But wait. How will simplifying my life help with my depression? Won't it just make things worse when I have to give things up? I'll just feel like a failure when I can't keep up, won't I? I suppose you could if you let it. But you learned how to dispute negative thoughts back on Day 4 and how to master your mind on Day 8. Use these skills should your thoughts start wandering in that direction.

Simplifying your life will help because excessive activity causes stress, fatigue, guilt, resentment, regret, and anger. Once these emotions set in, you are headed for trouble with depression. So if you are feeling overwhelmed with life, I suggest you learn how to simplify before it's too late. Don't let those physical and emotional symptoms take hold.

If they already have and you feel like your mind and body have gone on strike, you're probably already suffering from depression. Let's look at how you can tell.

Depression can result from many sources. Sometimes it's a lengthy sadness which you ignored. Other times, you may have untreated post-traumatic stress disorder (PTSD) following some difficult life event. Another explanation is a chemical imbalance in your brain. In any case, don't ignore it. You need to get help.

One in five people suffer with a mental illness such as depression.[3] If you participate in an activity with five or more people, it's a pretty good bet one of them is suffering right now. If it's not you, then who? That's why it's important for everyone to know all they can about depression – to help themselves and others.

The signs and symptoms of depression vary from one individual to the next. Some of the more common ones are:

- Feeling restless or withdrawn

- Unable to fall asleep, stay asleep, or both

- Constant fatigue or lack of energy

- Excessive desire to be alone

- Difficulty with focus or remembering things

- Unexplained irritability or anger

- Feeling sad, lonely, or teary-eyed

- Feelings of guilt, shame, or unworthiness

- Frequent thoughts of death or suicide

Any time you experience a combination of these symptoms for more than two weeks, it's time to contact a mental health professional. See Day 3 for more information about asking for help.

Process

It is important for you to self-monitor when it comes to mental health. Track your feelings, and know when you are on overload. How many symptoms are you currently experiencing? Did you realize they might be related? If you have several symptoms listed, how does it make you feel to know you might be suffering from depression? Does it bring relief or fear?

Do you allow your emotions to make decisions for you? Remember to make fact-based decisions. Don't say yes to something grudgingly. You will only resent doing it on an already overtaxed schedule. Also, remember to simplify and set boundaries. Get to know yourself, and know when it's time to reach out for help.

If you already suffer from depression, both you and your family need to learn more about it. A strong support team is critical when you are struggling with depression. Do your family and friends know you're suffering? Don't wait for them to ask if they can help; tell them what they can do to help you.

Engage

Depression Awareness. Knowledge is power. In this case, knowledge about depression gives you the power to make lifestyle changes which may help. Research some of the following sites to learn about depression signs, symptoms, treatments and self-help tips. Write down anything you want to remember in your journal.

- Sadness to Joy – https://sadnesstojoy.com/resources/help-for-depression

- Anxiety & Depression Association of America - http://bit.ly/2ddCwlV

- National Institute on Mental Health - http://bit.ly/2dIsxsP

- Healthline - http://bit.ly/2eoRre4

- National Alliance on Mental Illness - http://bit.ly/1C4kom2

- Depression and Bipolar Support Alliance - http://bit.ly/1mu3JUc

Be Inspired. Take time to read scripture, a devotional, or an inspirational book. Listen to uplifting music, and focus on the lyrics. Digest their meaning and how they inspire you.

Inspiration Suggestions

You largely constructed your depression. It wasn't given to you. Therefore, you can deconstruct it. Albert Ellis

> *That's the thing about depression: A human being can survive almost anything, as long as she sees the end in sight. But, depression is so insidious, and it compounds daily, that it's impossible to ever see the end. The fog is like a cage without a key. Elizabeth Wurtzel*
>
> *If you don't think your anxiety, depression, sadness and stress impact your physical health, think again. All of these emotions trigger chemical reactions in your body, which can lead to inflammation and a weakened immune system. Learn how to cope, sweet friend. There will always be dark days. Kris Carr*

Reflect

1. What did you think, talk, and post about today? Were you able to stay focused on the donut (it's okay to say no to something if it's what's best for your own health, knowledge is power and now you have it), or did you spend the day focused on the hole (you have to help everyone even if it's not healthy)?

2. How will you implement what you discovered today to help you find joy?

3. How do you feel about the idea of simplifying your life? Are you experiencing anxiety about what others will think if you step away from certain activities? Are you unsure how they will manage without you? What tools can you use to help ease these feelings and do what's best for you?

4. What symptoms were you able to identify in yourself? Were you surprised to learn you had so many? Did it bring you relief to know there's a name for what you're experiencing?

5. What did you learn about depression? How can you help yourself or others with this knowledge?

6. Do you need to go back and re-visit Day 3 and ask for some help?

7. Which of the Inspiration Suggestions did you choose? What stood out that you'd like to remember?

8. Go to https://sadnesstojoy.com/forum/21days, and share your thoughts about depression and mental illness.

Day 14: Get Your Sleep

This has been a long, hard journey. I've asked a lot from you mentally, physically and emotionally, and we've taken a few breaks to renew our spirit, but what about renewing our body? I think we should take today to rest and recharge.

———————

Saggy, baggy eyes, a slow gait, and sad appearance seem to be the norm in the morning. The first thing people say when you ask if they're okay is, "I didn't sleep well last night." Research shows more than 30% of the population suffers from insomnia (inability to get enough sleep).[1] But why do we have so much trouble sleeping?

Many times, insomnia is self-inflicted. Either we stay up too late, or we do things which prevent good sleep. I can't help if you stay up too late, but let's look at what might be affecting your sleep even when you do go to bed at a reasonable time.

- Medical illness – cold, flu, pain, heartburn, kidney problem, etc.

- Emotional upset – anxiety, depression, worry, anger, etc.

- Prescriptions – read labels carefully, and ask your doctor

- Caffeine overuse or consumption late in the day – coffee, tea, soda Note: Caffeine withdrawal can cause headaches, but stick with it, and they will subside.

- Alcohol consumption

- Eating a heavy meal before bed

- Taking naps

- Exercise or physical activity late in the day

- Electronics – TV, computer, smart phone, video games

- Sleep setting – temperature, strong colors, noise, comfort, etc.

- Irregular sleep schedule – going to bed at different times

Most people are not aware these things can affect their ability to fall asleep and stay asleep. If you are still skeptical, track your sleep. Record your activity and sleep patterns. You'll become a believer.

Each of us can control, for the most part, our sleep habits. If you've had children, you understand the importance of a bedtime routine. It wires your brain to understand the steps to take before sleep. Bath, book, bed, or something like that. My grandchildren all have a bedtime routine, and I've rarely seen them have trouble falling asleep. If it works for children, it will work for adults too. So let's set up a bedtime routine.

Start with setting a bedtime. Your daytime routine will dictate this. If you start work at 6:00 am and you live 30 minutes away, you need to get to bed earlier than someone who starts work at 8:30 am and lives 15 minutes away.

The Centers for Disease Control (CDC) indicates adults need between seven and eight hours of sleep per night.[2] So decide what time you need to get up, and subtract eight hours from that. This is your new bedtime.

Now decide on your bedtime activities. Avoid electronics of any kind in this plan. You may want to sit outside and gaze at the stars for a few minutes, then get dressed for bed, and brush your teeth. Once in bed, you like to read a book for 15-20 minutes, and then it's lights out. Whatever you decide, stick with it.

Habits are formed by repetition. The more you repeat your bedtime routine, the more likely you are to train your brain to sleep when it's time. Here are some great links for more information on sleep problems and suggestions for eliminating them.

- Centers for Disease Control (CDC) - http://bit.ly/1I50rj7

- Help Guide - http://bit.ly/10jc8kB

- Caring.com - http://bit.ly/1HmQRs9

Process

Do you have trouble sleeping? Which of the factors listed may be contributing? What can you do to eliminate, or at least lessen the impact, of whatever factors are affecting your sleep?

Use the links provided to find a solution. Now, plan to implement the changes one at a time to see which one works best for you. Did you find anything helpful on these sites? Which strategies can you use to help with your specific sleep problems?

Engage

Getting a good night's sleep often requires some effort. Tracking your sleep habits and planning to overcome obstacles will help.

A Good Night's Sleep. Create a Sleep Tracker using a calendar or the chart provided in your journal. Record your sleep habits for a week, and use the **PIRA** process to plan how you will implement better sleep habits the following week. Finally, implement your plan and record how it worked. Identify any patterns, and plan to address them.

Be Inspired. Take time to read scripture, a devotional, or an inspirational book. Listen to uplifting music, and focus on the lyrics. Digest their meaning and how they inspire you.

Inspiration Suggestions

Sorrow can be alleviated by good sleep, a bath and a glass of wine.
Thomas Aquinas

Sleep has been provided by nature to do the body's healing work, and it takes seven or eight hours for this process to happen. Commit to getting at least seven to eight hours of good quality sleep every night to keep your body and hormones in balance. Suzanne Somers

Then Jesus said, "Come to me, all of you who are weary and carry heavy burdens, and I will give you rest." Matthew 11:28 (NLT)

Reflect

1. What did you think, talk, and post about today? Were you able to stay focused on the donut (you can control how well you sleep, there are things you can do to help), or did you spend the day focused on the hole (no matter what you do, you just can't sleep)?

2. How will you implement what you discovered today to help you find joy?

3. What sleep problems have you experienced? What is your typical bedtime routine?

4. How do you feel about giving up your electronics later in the evening? What activity can you do instead?

5. How do you feel about giving up caffeine and alcohol later in the day? What can you drink instead?

6. What obstacles do you think might interfere with your ability to adopt healthier bedtime habits? How will you overcome them?

7. Which of the Inspiration Suggestions did you choose? What stood out that you'd like to remember?

8. Go to https://sadnesstojoy.com/forum/21days, and share your thoughts about developing a bedtime routine.

Day 15: Be Spontaneous

Were you able to get some rest? I hope so. It's hard to believe we've come such a long way and only have seven days left. It hasn't been easy, so you should be proud of what you've accomplished. Now let's celebrate and have some fun.

His bright eyes were filled with excitement. His little body just couldn't sit still. That pile was so big. It was almost scary but not enough to hold him back. No sir. That pile was filled with possibility, and he just couldn't contain his glee. Three, two, one, GO!

He ran with all his might as quickly as his snowsuit would allow and threw himself headlong into the huge pile of snow. Up he jumped, full of giggles squealing, "Again, again!"

Nothing could keep my son from that snow pile. He didn't care how ridiculous he looked bundled up from head to toe, or if he might get hurt. All he cared about was the fun which lay in front of him. He was four at the time and life was all about fun. He didn't think first about risks or consequences. He just did it.

We were all four once. So what happened? When did we lose the *life is about fun* mentality? More importantly, why did we lose it?

As we get older, people expect us to be more responsible. To weigh the risks, benefits, and consequences of our actions before we do anything. We're so busy deciding if we should do something, we never get around to doing it.

Well, that changes now! It's time to quit planning and worrying so much and learn to be more spontaneous.

I'm not suggesting you throw planning out the window permanently, or even on a consistent basis, but I am suggesting you have some fun when an opportunity arises. Just do something on the spur of the moment.

I'm also not suggesting you throw caution to the wind and start jumping off tall buildings, or take up sky diving without proper training and safety equipment. Sensibility rules.

With all that said, take advantage of opportunities when they arise. Here are a few suggestions to get you started.

- Build a sand castle, or bury yourself in the sand

- Build a snowman, or have a snowball fight

- Pick leaves, and make a collage

- Turn up the radio, and sing out loud

- Dance even when there's no dance floor

- Play in the rain, and stomp in puddles

- Camp out in the living room – turn off the power, use flashlights, build a tent with blankets, and eat campfire food

- Finger paint or color in a coloring book (they make adult themes)

- Clean a room in your house until it sparkles

- Get a manicure, pedicure or massage – just because

- Phone (not text or email) an old friend to say hello and catch up

These are just a few ideas to get you started. Now it's up to you. Think of things you enjoyed as a child, in your youth or as a young adult. Again, you aren't trying to turn into a child, just live life through the eyes of a child. With all the wonder and excitement life provided.

Process

Think through things you enjoyed doing when you were younger. Which have you thought about doing lately and talked yourself out of because you're too old or too ... whatever?

Engage

Seizing the moment is a skill we all need to learn, because having fun should be a priority in everyone's life.

Spur of the Moment. It's hard to plan to be spontaneous. I believe planning a spontaneous moment is an oxymoron. However, you can plan for things you'd like to do if an opportunity presents itself.

Use the Spur of the Moment sheet in your journal to gather ideas. Did anything from my list sound interesting? What things came to mind as you read which you'd like to try? What's something you've seen someone do and said, "they should know better" but secretly wished you were doing it with them? Or how about some things about which you've said, "I wish I had time to do that?"

Be Inspired. Take time to read scripture, a devotional, or an inspirational book. Listen to uplifting music, and focus on the lyrics. Digest their meaning and how they inspire you.

Inspiration Suggestions

Why? It's an excellent question. But an even better one is... Why not? Lara Whatley

A sign of inner peace is a tendency to think and act spontaneously rather than on fears based on past experiences. Dr. Bernie Siegel

The best time to plant a tree was 20 years ago. The second best time is now. Chinese Proverb

Reflect

1. What did you think, talk, and post about today? Were you able to stay focused on the donut (your life can be fun again) or did you spend the day focused on the hole (you're too old to have fun, what will people think if you do that)?

2. How will you implement what you discovered today to help you find joy?

3. What were your thoughts when you read the list of suggestions I made?

4. What obstacles would you need to overcome to do some of them? How will you overcome them?

5. How could you be more spontaneous?

6. Which of the Inspiration Suggestions did you choose? What stood out that you'd like to remember?

7. Go to https://sadnesstojoy.com/forum/21days, and share your thoughts about being more spontaneous.

Day 16: Energize Yourself

Did you enjoy yourself yesterday? Hopefully you allowed yourself to let loose a little. You may have discovered having fun takes energy you just don't have.

That's understandable. We've come a long way, and you may be starting to feel fatigued. Most road trips have rest stops along the way for just this purpose. However, resting is not what we need to do. Chances are you're doing too much of that already because you don't have the energy to do anything else. I see a recharging station up ahead. That's exactly what we need. Let's stop by and recharge our batteries, so we can get back to enjoying life.

========================

When people describe a heart attack, they say it feels like an elephant sitting on their chest. Have you ever felt like that, only all over your body? That's not a heart attack. That's fatigue. Every task seems overwhelming. Walking around, or even sitting upright, feels like you have a 100-lb weight around your neck.

Fatigue is very common in those suffering from anxiety and depression. That's one of the reasons people say they can't get out of bed. Or they complain getting cleaned up and dressed is too difficult. They're probably not lazy, they're suffering from stress- or depression-related fatigue.

Dr. Geisler, in a research review published in a 2014 edition of the Journal of Depression and Anxiety says, "Left untreated, fatigue can contribute to longer and more severe depression."[1]

There are ways to fight fatigue though. We talked about physical activity on Day 6 and sleep habits on Day 14. Being consistent in these two areas will certainly help with your fatigue. But here are some other suggestions.

- See your family doctor to rule out any medical cause

- Take up Yoga

- Balance your schedule with your body clock's sleep and wake cycle

- Lose weight

- Eat a healthy breakfast high in fiber, complex carbs, and protein

- Take a break – stand up, stretch, or walk around a bit

- Drink plenty of water

- Unplug or limit mindless electronics - do something mentally active instead

- Increase your B-vitamin intake – it helps fight stress

- Increase your D-vitamin intake – it helps fight depression

Process

Just because your fatigue is normal doesn't mean you should live with it. What can you do today to improve your habits to provide more energy? Pick something from the list, or come up with something on your own. Use the PIRA process to set goals and monitor your progress.

Engage

Create an Energy Plan. Using the template provided, develop an energy plan. Monitor when you feel fatigued. It could be related to diet or low activity level. For example, I usually crash after lunch. When I started eating a lighter lunch and taking more stretch breaks, my fatigue improved.

List three or four things you can do when fatigue comes on. Include a combination of physical activity to refresh your body and mental activity to renew your mind.

For example, one of Stephen Covey's seven habits is to *Sharpen the Saw*.[2] The premise is it takes you much longer to cut through a log with a dull-bladed saw than with a sharp one. If you would stop to sharpen your saw, it would cut more quickly, saving you time and energy in the long run.

Unfortunately, most people won't take time to sharpen the saw. They just keep pushing through. But fatigue eventually causes a lack of focus and mistakes. When you start feeling tired, find yourself reading something twice, or getting confused, take a break. Get up, and move around. It helps.

I highly recommend Stephen Covey's books. I've read them and attended training on how to implement the habits. They are invaluable to anyone wishing to change habits. I've provided a link to his page below.

- Seven Habits of Highly Effective People - http://bit.ly/1mvwAVf

Be Inspired. Take time to read scripture, a devotional, or an inspirational book. Listen to uplifting music, and focus on the lyrics. Digest their meaning and how they inspire you.

Inspiration Suggestions

Energy & persistence conquer all things. Benjamin Franklin

In times of great stress or adversity, it's always best to keep busy, to plow your anger and your energy into something positive. Lee Iacocca

Each time he said, "My grace is all you need. My power works best in weakness." So now I am glad to boast about my weaknesses, so that the power of Christ can work through me. 2 Corinthians 12:9 (NLT)

When you are enthusiastic about what you do, you feel this positive energy. It's very simple. Paulo Coelho

He gives power to the weak and strength to the powerless. Even youths will become weak and tired, and young men will fall in exhaustion. But those who trust in the Lord will find new strength. They will soar high on wings like eagles. They will run and not grow weary. They will walk and not faint. Isaiah 40:29-31 (NLT)

Reflect

1. What did you think, talk, and post about today? Were you able to stay focused on the donut (there are things you can do to fight your fatigue), or did you spend the day focused on the hole (you're always tired, it will never change, so why even try)?

2. How will you implement what you discovered today to help you find joy?

3. At what time of day does your energy start slipping away? What can you do to counteract that feeling?

4. Did you notice any patterns to when your fatigue comes on? What can you tweak in your routine to help fight it?

5. Which of the Inspiration Suggestions did you choose? What stood out that you'd like to remember?

6. Go to https://sadnesstojoy.com/forum/21days, and share your thoughts about ways to keep your energy level high.

Day 17: Increase Your Face-Time

Are you feeling stronger and more energized after our day at the recharging station? Did you make plans for how to have more energy for the rest of our journey? You'll need it if we're going to finish strong.

So far, it's just been the two of us traveling together, which is fine. I've truly enjoyed it and hope you are too. But today I thought we might add a friend or two. Things are always easier and more fun with friends around.

━━━━━━━━━━━━━━━

Facebook says I have 429 friends. I have 32 more on Twitter. Another 45 on Pinterest, and 23 on Instagram. Apparently, I have lots of friends. So why do I feel so lonely?

After all, that's a whole lot of friends. But how many of them do I know their favorite color or favorite sports team? How many would I call if I needed help? These people aren't friends; they're acquaintances.

A friend is someone you would call in the middle of the night if you needed help. They are someone you would get up in the middle of the night to go help. You would tell them your deepest, darkest secret and know for certain they would never tell anyone. Now let's count how many friends I have.

Social media has been phenomenal for sharing our life with others who are not nearby. However, it has also been the downfall of face-to-face relationships. We need less Facebook and more face-time.

Face-Time is how much time you spend physically face-to-face with someone. Online messages and posts can keep you in the loop, but for the most part, they are completely devoid of emotion. You can't tell through written words if someone is struggling emotionally or stressed at work. These are things only face-to-face encounters will reveal.

Life is not meant to be lived in isolation. That only feeds depression. We were meant to live in community. To do things together, with and for each other. As society moves farther and farther into the electronic world, we need to consciously and purposefully plan for more face-time.

Process

How many times have you said to someone, "we need to get together soon," only to say the same thing six months later? Believe me, I get it. We all lead busy lives. But if we don't purposefully plan face-time with others, it simply won't happen. So who do you need to start connecting with in person? How can you make that happen?

Engage

As a society, we've lost the personal touch. Everything happens electronically these days. You can counteract that by increasing your face-time.

Create a Face-Time Plan. Use a calendar or the sheet provided to set goals for yourself. Then plan a week's worth of activity. Start simple.

Name five friends or family members who live nearby you haven't spent face-time with in the past six months. Your first goal may be to meet one of them for a movie. That doesn't require a lot of conversation, so it's a good place to start if you're struggling. If it's improvement for you, it's perfect. Start there.

Others may already be leading a relatively normal lifestyle and just need to convert from electronic contact time to physical face-time. That's great. Plan to add one face-to-face activity each week. You may need to simplify or rearrange your schedule to make it happen, but it's worth it.

The point is to set goals and track your progress. Use the PIRA process or the Face-Time Tracker in your journal. Keep in mind, it's about progress, not perfection. Add a little more each week or so to keep yourself challenged.

Start a Friendship Circle. Make a list of 5 to 10 friends with whom you want to spend more face-time. Take turns planning a monthly activity together. Plan far enough out people won't already be booked up. It can be as simple as seeing a movie together or playing a game. Or you could go all out, get dressed up, and spend a night on the town.

Can't think of 5 to 10 friends? It's time to meet some new ones. Take a class, or start a new hobby. Join a reading, gardening, or travel club. Are you athletic? Join a team like bowling, tennis, or golf.

Be Inspired. Take time to read scripture, a devotional, or an inspirational book. Listen to uplifting music, and focus on the lyrics. Digest their meaning and how they inspire you.

Inspiration Suggestions

I'm tired of being inside my head. I want to live out here, with you. Colleen McCarty

We're all a part of this world, and it's up to us to make this one chance at living worthwhile. But the only way to do that is by doing it together. Robert Vanleeuwen

Two people are better off than one, for they can help each other succeed. If one person falls, the other can reach out and help. But someone who falls alone is in real trouble. Ecclesiastes 4:9-10 (NLT)

Song – Better Together by Jack Johnson*

*Video available at https://sadnesstojoy.com/inspiration/music

Reflect

1. What did you think, talk, and post about today? Were you able to stay focused on the donut (you've got friends, real ones, not just virtual ones), or did you spend the day focused on the hole (no one cares or has time for your problems, you're just a burden on everyone)?

2. How will you implement what you discovered today to help you find joy?

3. Think about the five friends you listed earlier whom you haven't seen in six months. What's stopping you from spending face-time with them? What would it take to change that?

4. Is there someone you need to forgive before you can re-connect? How about someone you need to apologize to before you can re-connect? What's stopping you? Find a way to make this happen sooner rather than later.

5. How does the idea of meeting with friends make you feel? Why?

6. What obstacles would you need to overcome to make these interactions more comfortable? How will you overcome them?

7. Did you have trouble coming up with a list of 5 to 10 friends? What did you decide to do to meet new friends?

8. Which of the Inspiration Suggestions did you choose? What stood out that you'd like to remember?

9. Go to https://sadnesstojoy.com/forum/21days, and share your thoughts about spending more face-time with others.

Day 18: Explore New Interests

Isn't it refreshing to get out and meet with friends? It always makes me feel better. I hope it did for you as well. Now that we've got some friends along for the journey, let's try something new. Trying new things is never as scary when you've got a friend along.

―――――――――

The backpack sat by the door. New, neatly pressed clothes lay ready to wear. The smell of bacon and eggs filled the house. Everything was perfect. The excitement of the first day of school couldn't be matched.

However, the anxiety it brought hid somewhere inside. What would my teacher be like? Would I know anyone in class? What if I did something wrong and looked stupid? What if people laughed at me? What if no one wanted to sit with me at lunch? It seemed our entire future hinged on how that one day went.

Somewhere between kindergarten and 12th grade we lost our love for learning. We decided not knowing something was uncool. Admitting we needed help was the social kiss of death. And wearing the wrong thing, or being seen with the wrong friend, was an immediate trip into social exile.

It's time we re-ignite our love for learning. Start by being willing to admit you don't know something. Go someplace where no one knows you if that helps, but make a commitment to learn something new. Take a class, start a hobby, or research something you find interesting.

You'll still face some of the anxiety of meeting new people and trying something new. That can't be avoided. But the joy of accomplishing something new far outweighs the momentary discomfort.

Here are some activities you might want to try.

- Play a new game

- Cook a new dish

- Dine at a new restaurant

- Take an improv class (scary, I know, but it's fun)

- Research a cause which tugs at your heart

- Sew, knit, quilt, fish, hunt, or camp

- Take up photography

Process

Learning something new serves multiple purposes. It gets us out of isolation and connects us with others. It's physically and mentally engaging. And mastering a new skill provides a sense of accomplishment. What's something new you'd like to learn more about?

Engage

This activity will be one of the most difficult, because it requires you to be vulnerable. You've worked hard to feel good about yourself only to now admit you don't know something. Combine that with the new relationship skills we worked on yesterday and you've got a complete double whammy. It may be tough, but muster up some courage and give it a try.

Short-Term Bucket List. Make a list of 10 activities you would enjoy. Don't worry about cost, time, or talent. Just list them. Now pick one, and make it happen. Schedule time this week to either do it or start the planning process. Keep working until you get through the list.

Be Inspired. Take time to read scripture, a devotional, or an inspirational book. Listen to uplifting music, and focus on the lyrics. Digest their meaning and how they inspire you.

Inspiration Suggestions

By making yourself a life-long learner you'll keep discovering new and exciting things about yourself and others. Rachel Robins

Always walk through life as if you have something new to learn, and you will. Vernon Howard

You can learn new things at any time in your life if you're willing to be a beginner. If you actually learn to like being a beginner, the whole world opens up to you. Barbara Sher

Intelligent people are always ready to learn. Their ears are open for knowledge. Proverbs 18:15 (NLT)

Reflect

1. What did you think, talk, and post about today? Were you able to stay focused on the donut (learning can be fun, the reward really is worth the risk), or did you spend the day focused on the hole (you're too old to learn new things, people will laugh at you when you don't do it right)?

2. How will you implement what you discovered today to help you find joy?

3. Did you have a hard time coming up with 10 things you would enjoy doing? Why do you think that is?

4. How did you feel about trying something new? What activity did you select to do? Why did you choose that one? Is it comfortable or a challenge?

5. Did you face any fear about your choice of activity? Did you overcome your fear and take the first step towards making it happen?

6. Which of the Inspiration Suggestions did you choose? What stood out that you'd like to remember?

7. Go to https://sadnesstojoy.com/forum/21days, and share your thoughts about trying something new.

Day 19: Help Others

Yesterday we learned to take some chances and try new things. Did you push through your fears and try something new? Hopefully it was at least a little bit enjoyable. And the good news is, it will get easier each time you do it.

So far, this journey has been all about us. We've been focused on how to help ourselves. But look, up ahead, someone's fallen under the weight of their journey. I think we're strong enough now to maybe offer some help. What do you think? Let's at least try. Even if we can't help, we can give them a smile and some encouragement. Sometimes, that's enough.

———————————

As I pulled up to the drive-thru window, I reached out to hand the cashier my card. She smiled as she handed me the bag filled with my favorite drive-thru meal and said, "Have a nice day. Your order was taken care of by the person ahead of you." Did they recognize me? No. They would have waved or pulled over to say hi. Then I realized a total stranger just paid for my lunch. Wow. That doesn't happen very often.

That small act of kindness made my day. I couldn't stop thinking about it. You can create that same feeling for others. Here are a few ways to show kindness to others:

- Hold the door for someone

- Volunteer at a shelter

- Bake something special for a neighbor or coworker

- Donate gently-used items to a thrift store

- Let someone with fewer items, small children, or elderly go in front of you at the checkout line

- Mow someone's grass who is sick or out of town

- Prepare a meal for someone who is sick or has a family member in the hospital. Better yet, bring a meal to the hospital if their diet allows.

- Let another car cut in front of you in the pick-up line at school

- Visit a sick person in the hospital or elderly person in a care facility

- Pay a compliment to a total stranger

- Smile at someone for no reason

- Volunteer for an organization whose passion you share

Think of small ways to help someone. They don't have to take time or money. When you help someone in need it helps put your concerns in perspective, because doing for others also helps us feel good about ourselves.

Process

No one wants to ask for help. Sometimes we don't even know we need it. But kindness is always appreciated. What could someone do to make you feel better in a time of need? If it would help you, it would probably help them as well. What things from the list could you start doing for others? What are some unique ways you could help others based on your strengths?

Engage

It's easy to think about doing something but a little more difficult to do it. So stretch yourself and try it.

Acts of Kindness. Create a list on a 3x5 card of simple ways you could help someone or show kindness. Keep it with you. Whenever you feel yourself sliding into stress, anxiety, or depression, pull out that card and do something for someone else. It will give you an instant pick me up by getting your focus off your needs and onto someone else's. There's that donut again.

When we're struggling, we don't see all our blessings. In *This is the Stuff,* Francesca Battistelli reminds us how easy it is to forget the many ways we are blessed when we are in the middle of our own struggles. All we can see is what's going wrong.

We can help others because we have something they need. No matter how bad you feel you can always give a smile or hug. It could be time, money, physical ability, or a skill, but you have something they don't. Find out what it is, and give generously. They'll feel better and so will you.

Be Inspired. Take time to read scripture, a devotional, or an inspirational book. Listen to uplifting music, and focus on the lyrics. Digest their meaning and how they inspire you.

Inspiration Suggestions

Kindness costs nothing, but it's value is priceless. Unknown

Kindness is not an act. It is a lifestyle. Anthony Douglas

The best way to cheer yourself up is to try to cheer somebody else up. Mark Twain

If you want happiness for an hour — take a nap. If you want happiness for a day — go fishing. If you want happiness for a year — inherit a fortune. If you want happiness for a lifetime — help someone else. Chinese Proverb

Dear children, let's not merely say that we love each other; let us show the truth by our actions. 1 John 3:18 (NLT)

Reflect

1. What did you think, talk, and post about today? Were you able to stay focused on the donut (you may not be where you want to be, but you're better off than where you were and you're better off than a lot of others), or did you spend the day focused on the hole (you don't have anything to share with others, besides they don't have it as bad as you do, you've got to get better first)?

2. How will you implement what you discovered today to help you find joy?

3. Could you relate to the opening story? What would you do if that was you? How would it make you feel?

4. What are some ways you can think of to help others? What obstacles would need to be overcome for you to go do it?

5. Which of the Inspiration Suggestions did you choose? What stood out that you'd like to remember?

6. Go to https://sadnesstojoy.com/forum/21days, and share your thoughts about helping others.

Day 20: Enhance Your Spiritual Life

Wow! That felt good to help someone, didn't it? Thinking about others and their needs really does help get your mind off your own problems.

Did you know God's plan is for us to love others and help them? We're almost finished with our journey, and we've made good time. So let's take it easy today and just spend some time with God. We've learned a lot about each other on this journey, because we've spent so much time together. In the same way, we can learn so much more about God if we just spend a little time with him. Let's carve out some time today.

Children grow up quickly. They crawl and walk in the blink of an eye. Next is preschool and then the first day of kindergarten arrives. Before you know it, *Pomp and Circumstance* escorts them across the stage for their diploma.

Physical growth seems to happen without any effort. Intellectual growth, on the other hand, requires time and energy. Now let's look at spiritual growth.

Men and women of faith often believe all it takes to be spiritually mature is a decision, baptism, first communion or bar mitzvah. But that is only partially true. While these events are important to your spiritual growth journey, they are simply points on a map along the way, like that first day of kindergarten and graduation stage.

Spiritual growth, just like intellectual growth, requires a commitment of time and energy. It starts with a desire to learn more about your journey. What does it really mean to be a Christian? Or Jewish? Or Muslim?

I'm a Christian, so I can only speak to that journey. If you practice another faith, some of the same principles apply, however, the terms will be different.

What does a spiritual growth journey require?

- **Desire** – to learn new things about God and get to know him

- **Study of the Bible** – God's guidebook for our lives

- **Prayer** – a way to communicate with God

- **Worship** – an opportunity to thank God for his blessings

- **Repentance** – sorrow for our sins and attempts to improve

- **Giving** – providing our time, talent, and money for God's church

- **Service** – helping others with our time, talent, and money

The spiritual growth journey doesn't end until we die. We will continue to grow and become spiritually mature if we strive to do these seven things better each day. Will you join me on this journey?

Process

Are you currently practicing some form of faith-based worship? If so, does it give you a sense of peace? If not, consider using the seven areas of growth listed above to go deeper. Which area would be the best place for you to start? Why? What could you do in that area to start growing?

Engage

Begin planning your journey to spiritual maturity today.

Create a Spiritual Growth Plan. Use the PIRA process to record your goals and track your progress in each of the areas listed above. It can be as simple as deciding to attend a local church service. You may already do that but want to spend more time in Bible study or serving others. It's a personal decision. Remember, progress, not perfection.

Be Inspired. Take time to read scripture, a devotional, or an inspirational book. Listen to uplifting music, and focus on the lyrics. Digest their meaning and how they inspire you.

Inspiration Suggestions

As pressure and stress bear down on me, I find joy in your commands. Psalms 119:143 (NLT)

I will never forget your commandments, for you have used them to restore my joy and health. Psalms 119: 93 (NLT)

Physical training is good, but training for godliness is much better, promising benefits in this life and in the life to come. 1 Timothy 4:8 (NLT)

Spend your time and energy in training yourself for spiritual fitness. Physical exercise has some value, but spiritual exercise is much more important for it promises a reward in both this life and the next. This is true and everyone should accept it. 1 Timothy 4:7-9 (NLT)

I may be down, but I am not out. If I return to God, he will accept my repentant prayer and restore me. Hosea 14:1-2 (paraphrase)

Song – Word of God Speak by MercyMe*

Song – Praise You in this Storm by Casting Crowns*

Song – Eye of the Storm by Ryan Stephenson*

Song – Thy Will by Hilary Scott & the Scott Family*

*Video available at https://sadnesstojoy.com/inspiration/music

Reflect

1. What did you think, talk, and post about today? Were you able to stay focused on the donut (God has a purpose for your suffering and it's not too late to build a relationship and have Him help you get through it), or did you spend the day focused on the hole (you don't need God, he hasn't helped you so far, why should you trust him now)?

2. How will you implement what you discovered today to help you find joy?

3. If you had to assess your status on the spiritual growth journey, which phrase best describes you? Why?

   o   I didn't even know there was a trip planned

   o   I'm just starting out

   o   I'm along for the ride

   o   I'm making steady progress

   o   I'm leading the troops

4. What would your next step be on this journey?

5. What obstacles might prevent you from taking that next step? How will you overcome them?

6. Which of the Inspiration Suggestions did you choose? What stood out that you'd like to remember?

7. Go to https://sadnesstojoy.com/forum/21days, and share your thoughts about spiritual growth and the habits it requires.

Day 21: Pick Your Battles

Can you believe it? We made it! This is our last day together. That may bring feelings of joy, but it may also bring feelings of fear and sadness. Don't worry though. I've watched you as we've walked this road together. You're stronger now. You've got this. You don't need me any longer, so go on now. Get out there and finish up this last stretch. Then go conquer the world and enjoy every minute of it!

⸺

As we come to the end of our 21-day journey, let's focus on our Donut Dare again. Each day we addressed a different area of wellness to help you change your focus from what's missing to what you have. How did you do? Were you able to make positive changes in your life? I certainly hope so.

Now, look back through each day, and grade yourself. Give yourself an A, B, C, D or F for each day. If you skipped any days because you were already healthy in that area, that's fine. Just give it an NA for not applicable. Next, write down any area where you scored a D or an F.

Grades like that mean it's time for a refresher course. Reflect on those days, and decide why you weren't successful at mastering the ideas or skills. Use the **PIRA** process, and plan to tackle those again. Continue this process until you have mastered them.

Now it's time to pick your battles. You can't have everything, so do you want to fight for a joy-filled life or fight for the comfort zone where you've been living? If you want to fight for that joy, it will require you to leave some things behind. But what will they be?

Over the next few days, list the five most important things in your life. Use the **PIRA** process, and plan to find joy in these five areas. You will need to consciously abandon other things that didn't make the list, and that's not always easy. It will require one of the three things I mentioned up front – an all-in commitment.

Are you totally committed to living a life of joy? Once you've made up your mind to have a joy-filled life at all cost, you'll have the strength and courage it will take to leave some things behind. If you have made that decision, it's time to trade your sorrows in for joy.

Process

I've introduced 21 areas of wellness where positive changes will lead to more joy. How did you do? What grade would you give yourself on your Wellness Journey? Remember, changing habits takes time. Don't get discouraged.

According to our definition in the beginning, joy is a deep feeling or condition of happiness or contentment. My prayer is that you have started developing habits which will help you find happiness and be content as you continue this journey. Thanks for taking it with me.

Engage

As we return to the Donut Dare where we started, I'd like to issue two challenges. The Donut Dare asked you to focus on all you have rather than all that's missing. These challenges will help you do just that.

30-Day Electronics Challenge. For the next 30 days, turn off or limit any electronics which don't lead to a positive focus. For instance, I used to be addicted to watching the news every morning as I got ready for work. I confess, I was addicted to the TODAY show. But have you watched the news lately? It's enough to depress anyone. So I quit. Cold turkey.

Instead, I found a Bible teaching by Joyce Meyer, whom I love. It just happens to be on while I'm getting ready. You might find a positive show which isn't faith-based on one of the home renovation channels, or a cooking channel. Stroll through the channel guide, and I'm sure you'll find something. I feel certain removing the negativity you're absorbing on TV and video games will help you feel better.

Now let's talk about those pesky cell phones. Talk about a mind-numbing waste of time. I understand the need to make phone calls, send emails, and texts. I even understand checking your bank balance or the weather. What I don't understand is the obsession with games and social media.

Now if you can honestly describe their positive impact, don't let me stop you. However, if you are chasing animals, matching candy, earning coins of any kind, or finding out what Aunt Sally is doing for the 12th time today, it's time to take a break. It's only for 30 days. I promise you can do it if you try.

When I took this challenge, I limited myself to 15 minutes of social media time each night. I can assure you if Aunt Sally breaks a hip or inherits a million dollars, you'll find out some other way or it can wait until the end of the day. I've drifted back into checking several times a day, so I guess it's time for me to start limiting my time again. Or I could get drastic and remove social media apps from my phone. But I think I'll start with limiting my time.

What will you do with all that time you ask? Work on your goals, get some physical activity, take up a new hobby, have dinner with a friend, meet with a support person or spend a little time on your spiritual growth journey. Haven't you been paying attention for the last 21 days?

30-Day Music Challenge. This challenge is like the Electronics Challenge, only it involves musical choices. My husband is a musician, so I certainly understand the need for music in your life. I'm not asking you to give up music completely for 30 days. I'm just asking you to make positive music choices.

There are a ton of *positive hits* radio stations locally and on the Internet. They come in all different genres of music. You can also find jazz or blues instrumental stations. Find something you like with a positive message. It may require some research, but the effort will pay off.

My local station has listeners from around the globe via the Internet. How do I know that? They are listener supported, meaning no commercials. During their fall fundraiser, people responded from around the world.

I've listened solely to Z88.3 radio for the past 20+ years. It is a top 40 kind of station, which bores my musician husband, but I love it. By hearing the same music repeatedly, I'm able to allow the words to sink in. I can sing along as loud as I want. The words of some of those songs have comforted me in times of trouble because they were so deeply ingrained in my heart.

Again, it's only for 30 days. You'll survive. You may even decide you like it. Besides, what have you got to lose?

Here are links to my favorite station and the sister stations they broadcast.

- Z88.3 – Positive Hits Safe for the Little Ears - http://zradio.org/

- G106.3 - Orlando's Gospel Music - http://www1.zradio.org/stream.php?sid=G

- Hot 95.9 – Positive Hip Hop and R&B - http://www1.zradio.org/stream.php?sid=H

- 103.7 The Rock – Positive Rock Alternative - http://www1.zradio.org/stream.php?sid=R

Be Inspired. Take time to read scripture, a devotional, or an inspirational book. Listen to uplifting music, and focus on the lyrics. Digest their meaning and how they inspire you.

Inspiration Suggestions

Life is short, so do what makes you happy, be with who makes you smile, laugh as much as you breathe, and love as long as you live. Rachel Ann Nunes

A very serious symptom of inner peace is a loss of ability to worry.
Dr. Bernie Siegel

There are more things to alarm us than to harm us, and we suffer more often in apprehension than reality. Seneca

See everyone else as enlightened except you. That means everyone you meet can teach you something. If they annoy or frustrate you, you can learn patience. Try to find the life lesson in everything and everyone you encounter. Focusing on the life lesson allows you to work on positive change, which will make you feel empowered instead of deflated. Richard Carlson

So don't worry about tomorrow, for tomorrow will bring its own worries. Today's trouble is enough for today. Matthew 6:34 (NLT)

Can all your worries add a single moment to your life? Luke 12:25 (NLT)

Song – Trading My Sorrows *by Darrell Evans**

*Video available at *https://sadnesstojoy.com/inspiration/music*

Reflect

1. What did you think, talk, and post about today? Were you able to stay focused on the donut (you've come so far, you may not be where you want to be yet, but you're not where you started), or did you spend the day focused on the hole (you've tried everything I've said, but nothing worked)?

2. How will you implement what you discovered today to help you find joy?

3. What are your thoughts about the Electronics Challenge? Are you up for it?

4. What obstacles might you face with this challenge? How will you overcome them?

5. What are your thoughts about the Music challenge? Are you up for it?

6. What obstacles might you face with this challenge? How will you overcome them?

7. Which of the Inspiration Suggestions did you choose? What stood out that you'd like to remember?

8. Go to https://sadnesstojoy.com/forum/21days, and share your thoughts about your Electronics Challenge or Music Challenge experience.

Documenting Your Journey

The remainder of this book is filled with pages where you will document your journey to a joy-filled life. This journal includes **Process** questions which will check for understanding and assess your current situation, **Engage** activities to practice new habits and build strength, and **Reflect** questions to guide your growth. These cover five areas of strength needed to live the joy-filled life. You may only need help in one or two areas. You may need help in all five.

- Mental Wellness – Days 1, 3, 4, 8, and 12

- Physical Wellness – Days 2, 6, 14, and 16

- Spiritual Wellness – Days 5, 10, 19, and 20

- Emotional Wellness – Days 7, 9, 15, 17, and 18

- Wellness Action Plan – Days 11, 13, and 21

Whatever your situation, the questions and activities in this journal are where change begins.

*Make copies of journal pages as needed.

Day 1 Process Activities

Have you ever thought about how many things you have which others around the world don't? Have you ever visited a homeless shelter or a food pantry? Each of us has people nearby without many of the simple comforts we take for granted. How can you make yourself more aware of those in your community who go without these things?

Day 1 Reflect Activities

What did you think, talk, and post about today? Were you able to stay focused on the donut (your blessings, what's going right), or did you spend the day focused on the hole (your misfortune, what's going wrong)?

What will you need to do to learn to be content with what you have?

How will you implement what you discovered today to help you find joy?

What did you feel when you thought about the homeless near you who have so little? What did you learn through this exercise?

Were you able to draw a clear line between wants and needs? How did it make you feel to realize so many things you thought were needs are really wants?

How many blessings were you able to add to your box? What were your thoughts when you realized how truly blessed you were?

Which of the Inspiration Suggestions did you choose? What stood out that you'd like to remember?

Go to https://sadnesstojoy.com/forum/21days, and share your thoughts about counting your blessings.

Day 2 Process Activities

What did you learn about healthy eating? Learning to eat healthy is a process. Knowledge is the first step. Next is implementation. Were you aware your dietary choices could be affecting how you feel emotionally? The food you eat could be affecting your level of joy. Dr. Joseph Mercola says, "Whether you need a quick pick-me-up or you've been struggling with poor mood for a while, the best place to start to turn your mood around is likely not in your medicine cabinet but right in your pantry or refrigerator."[4]

Day 2 - Meal Plan

Sun					
Sat					
Fri					
Thurs					
Wed					
Tues					
Mon					

Day 2 Reflect Activities

What did you think, talk, and post about today? Were you able to stay focused on the donut (the many healthy food choices you can eat), or did you spend the day focused on the hole (all the food choices you shouldn't eat, including actual donuts)?

How you will implement what you discovered today to help you find joy?

What did you learn about healthy eating? What improvements could you make to your current eating habits?

What changes are necessary based on your food tracking? What will you do differently?

What obstacles will you need to overcome to follow healthier eating habits? How will you overcome them?

Which of the Inspiration Suggestions did you choose? What stood out that you'd like to remember?

Go to https://sadnesstojoy.com/forum/21days, and share your thoughts about how food affects your mood.

Day 3 Process Activities

What were your thoughts when I asked if you were an independence addict? Do you have a hard time asking for help? The following links are some of my favorite sites which clarify mental health professionals' roles, what help is available, how you can find it, and some self-help resources.

- National Alliance on Mental Illness (NAMI) – http://bit.ly/V1KdCa

- National Institute of Mental Health (NIH) – http://bit.ly/2eTPLNe

- Anxiety & Depression Association of America (ADAA) – http://bit.ly/2ddCwlV

- Suicide Prevention Lifeline – http://bit.ly/1lYmABO

- Sadness to Joy – https://sadnesstojoy.com/resources/help-for-depression

Day 3 Reflect Activities

What did you think, talk, and post about today? Were you able to stay focused on the donut (help is available to you), or did you spend the day focused on the hole (you're all alone and no one understands)?

How will you implement what you discovered today to help you find joy?

Do you want to feel better, even if it means hard work and talking about how you got to where you are today? Are you willing to explore why you feel the way you do, even if it means digging into your past?

How does the term Mental Illness make you feel? Can you live with the stigma?

Which of the Inspiration Suggestions did you choose? What stood out that you'd like to remember?

Go to https://sadnesstojoy.com/forum/21days, and share your thoughts about asking for help.

Day 4 Process Activities

There are more ways to bully yourself than just the six I listed. Take time to think about each of these. As the victim of your own bullying, which ones do you allow to affect you? Which ones are the hot buttons your bully knows he can push to upset you? Why do they have the power to control you that way?

- Feel like everything is black or white

- Feel like it's all or nothing

- Feel like you should or shouldn't do something

- Feel responsible for things outside your control

- Jump to conclusions

- Filter out the good

Day 4 – Think Positive

Negative Thought	Positive Thought
1	1
2	2
3	3
4	4
5	5
6	6
7	7
8	8
9	9
10	10

Day 4 Reflect Activities

What did you think, talk, and post about today? Were you able to stay focused on the donut (your strengths and positive traits), or did you spend the day focused on the hole (your weaknesses, mistakes, and negative traits)?

How will you implement what you discovered today to help you find joy?

How do you bully yourself with your self-talk? Write down 10 negative self-talk statements, and rephrase them into positive affirmations.

Which of the Inspiration Suggestions did you choose? What stood out that you'd like to remember?

Go to https://sadnesstojoy.com/forum/21days, and share what you think about bullying yourself with your negative thoughts.

Day 5 Process Activities

In times of crisis, who do you call on for help? A friend? A family member? Or God?

Faith-based decisions are very personal. Not everyone believes in God, or even a higher power. They believe everything happens by chance. Is that you right now? All I ask today is to consider the possibility there is a God. That's it. I'm not asking you to make any public proclamation of faith. Just consider it.

If you are strong in your faith, lean on it in times of trouble.

However, if you aren't sure about all this, I urge you to learn more. There are some great books out there on the Christian faith. I would highly recommend you read *The Case for Faith: A Journalist Investigates the Toughest Objections to Christianity,*[1] or *The Case for Christ: A Journalist's Personal Investigation of the Evidence for Jesus,*[2] both by Lee Strobel.

Author's Note: Additional resources providing insight into Christianity can be found on my website at https://sadnesstojoy.com/resources/bible-study-scripture.

Day 5 – Explore Creation

Are the things we see in nature by chance or from God

Why do you think you feel that way?

Day 5 Reflect Activities

What did you think, talk, and post about today? Were you able to stay focused on the donut (there is a God in control even when things seem out of control), or did you spend the day focused on the hole (you're on your own when circumstances are out of control)?

How will you implement what you discovered today to help you find joy?

Will the knowledge God may be real change how you deal with crisis or uncertain times in your life? Why or why not?

Which of the Inspiration Suggestions did you choose? What stood out that you'd like to remember?

Go to https://sadnesstojoy.com/forum/21days, and share your thoughts about faith and how it provides support in times of trouble.

Day 6 Process Activities

How would you rate your current level of physical activity? Are there physical limitations preventing you from being more physically active? If so, are they limitations you can overcome, or will you need to think outside the box when planning physical activity? Just a hint, weight CAN be overcome? Yes, it takes time and effort, but it can be overcome? Disease and disability are things which would require outside-the-box thinking. Here are a few fitness sites offering ideas for everything from a seated chair workout for those with limited mobility to a full-blown boot camp. You can also find goal-setting advice and fitness tracking apps.

- Mayo Clinic - http://mayocl.in/1W4oV4M

- Spark People - http://bit.ly/2dSzQPo

- Fitness Magazine - http://bit.ly/2eaSgcE

- Map My Fitness - http://bit.ly/1DnTfdG

What's holding you back?

Day 6 - Physical Activity Plan – Activity 1

Have you seen a doctor recently for a physical to make sure you are healthy enough for physical activity? If not, schedule an appointment today.

What is your current level of daily physical activity?

What is your daily goal for your first week?

What activity have you chosen? Why?

What equipment, if any, is needed?

Will you do it alone or with a friend? Why?

What are your feelings about adding more physical activity?

What obstacles might you face? How will you overcome them?

Day 6 - Physical Activity Plan – Activity 2

Sun					
Sat					
Fri					
Thurs					
Wed					
Tues					
Mon					

Day 6 - Physical Activity Plan – Activity 3

Date: _____

What was your goal for today?

Did you meet it? Why or Why not?

Did you make it a priority, or did you make excuses? Why?

What obstacles did you face? How will you overcome them?

What might you do differently if you were to set this as a goal again?

Day 6 Reflect Activities

What did you think, talk, and post about today? Were you able to stay focused on the donut (you can feel better just by being more active), or did you spend the day focused on the hole (nothing will make you feel better so why try)?

How will you implement what you discovered today to help you find joy?

How do you currently stay active and healthy?

What goals have you set for yourself? Are they comfortable or challenging?

What obstacles will you need to overcome to be more physically active? How will you overcome them?

Which of the Inspiration Suggestions did you choose? What stood out that you'd like to remember?

Go to https://sadnesstojoy.com/forum/21days, and share your thoughts about adding more physical activity to your life.

Day 7 Process Activities

Living a life you don't enjoy is entirely within your control to change. It takes effort, but you can learn to enjoy life again. Start by changing one thing. Then add others as you feel comfortable. Think about some things you used to do but don't anymore. Really think about it. What makes you happy? What do you enjoy doing?

Day 7 – Things I Enjoy

Things I Would Enjoy	Things I Do Well
1	1
2	2
3	3
4	4
5	5
6	6
7	7
8	8
9	9
10	10

Day 7 – Happy Holidays

Things I Used to Enjoy About the Holidays	Things I Could Do to Enjoy the Holidays Again
1	1
2	2
3	3
4	4
5	5
6	6
7	7
8	8
9	9
10	10

Day 7 Reflect Activities

What did you think, talk, and post about today? Were you able to stay focused on the donut (living a life you enjoy is within your control), or did you spend the day focused on the hole (your life is miserable and there's nothing you can do to change it)?

How will you implement what you discovered today to help you find joy?

What area of your life do you feel negatively affects your emotions? Why?

What could you do to start enjoying that aspect of your life more?

What obstacles will you need to overcome to begin enjoying it? How will you overcome them?

Did you have a hard time listing 10 things you would enjoy and 10 things you feel you do well? Why do you think that is?

Which of the Inspiration Suggestions did you choose? What stood out that you'd like to remember?

Go to https://sadnesstojoy.com/forum/21days, and share your thoughts about learning to enjoy life.

Day 8 Process Activities

Learning to be more aware of your thoughts and emotions takes time and practice. Simplifying your life, which we'll talk about on Day 13, will help. By lessening your obligations, you'll free up your mind to focus on things that matter.

For instance, what activities are you doing right now only to make someone else happy? It's time to gracefully bow out. Just let them know you'll be stepping back for a while to focus on other obligations.

Remember the 12 other problems and emotions I mentioned your brain was distracted by earlier? Figure out how to let them go, because the less you do, the less you have to worry about. And spending less time worrying will free your brain up to better manage your current actions, thoughts, and emotions.

So think about it for a minute. What actions, thoughts or emotions are keeping you from a joy-filled life? Which one, if changed, would have the greatest impact? Let's start there.

Day 8 – PIRA Goal Sheet

PLAN – set goals, and map out steps to achieve them. Consider all obstacles which may interfere, and plan how you will overcome them.

IMPLEMENT – carry out your plan step-by-step. If an unplanned obstacle come up, use the strategies you developed in your plan. If an obstacle comes up you didn't plan for, pause to think before you respond.

REFLECT – at the end of each goal period (day/week/month), reflect on your plan. Did it go the way you hoped? If not, why. Did it go better than you hoped? Great! Why do you think that was the case?

ADJUST – change whatever didn't go the way you hoped. The unexpected obstacle, for instance. Plan how you will overcome it should it come up again.

Month: _____

What is your goal for this month? By what date will you complete it? Record it on that day of the month on your calendar.

What smaller steps will it take to meet this monthly goal? Record these on the last day of the week where you plan to accomplish it.

What smaller steps will it take to meet this weekly goal? Record these on the day of that week where you plan to accomplish them. Don't forget to make a specific appointment time rather than just list it on that day.

What obstacles might you face with this goal? How will you overcome them?

Day 8 – Pick Two

Date: _____

Pick two goals to achieve today unrelated to your monthly goal.

1.

2.

What advance preparation, smaller steps, or obstacles need to be considered to accomplish this goal today?

Day 8 Reflect Activities

What did you think, talk, and post about today? Were you able to stay focused on the donut (tomorrow can be better than today if you will just think about what didn't go well today and make small changes when you try again tomorrow), or did you spend the day focused on the hole (things will never change, you don't have the willpower or discipline to change, it's just too hard)?

How will you implement what you discovered today to help you find joy?

How does it make you feel to think about setting goals? Why do you think you feel that way?

What obstacles will you need to overcome to use the **PIRA** process? How will you overcome them?

What did you set for your first monthly goal? Did you have trouble breaking it down into smaller steps? Remember, it does get easier, so don't give up.

How did you do with your daily goals? What can you do differently to help you be more successful?

Which of the Inspiration Suggestions did you choose? What stood out that you'd like to remember?

Go to https://sadnesstojoy.com/forum/21days, and share your thoughts about self-awareness and tracking your progress toward positive habit changes.

Day 9 Process Activities

When my father passed away, I made something called a memory card. I created a postcard size sheet with one line on it – *My favorite memory of Jimmy is....* That's it. We handed these cards out at the visitation and funeral. Then, my daughter collected the completed ones in a basket. Over the next few days, those memories from childhood friends, coworkers, and distant relatives gave us a new understanding of my dad. We saw him through a fresh set of eyes. Those memory cards still bring me joy today.

What happy times do you remember? How does it make you feel when you recall them? Don't wait until someone is gone to discover all the interesting things about them. Ask now. Share your stories, and listen to theirs. It will bring a smile to your face and maybe, just maybe, a good mood-boosting belly laugh will well up and fall out.

Day 9 – I Like Myself

Things I Like About Myself	
1	9
2	10
3	11
4	12
5	13
6	14
7	15
8	

Things I Don't Like About Myself	
1	3
2	

I will work on changing #_____ above by doing the following:

Day 9 – Three Good Things

Good Things That Happened Today	
What Happened this Morning?	What Made It Good?
What Happened this Afternoon?	What Made It Good?
What Happened this Evening?	What Made It Good?

Day 9 Reflect Activities

What did you think, talk, and post about today? Were you able to stay focused on the donut (all the happy times you've had), or did you spend the day focused on the hole (all the unhappy things that have happened throughout your life or are happening right now)?

How will you implement what you discovered today to help you find joy?

What does happiness mean to you? What would it look like in your life?

Think about three happy memories from your childhood or earlier adult life. What makes them memorable? Why did they make you happy? Could you re-create them?

What can you do today to start recording your happy memories to look back on later?

Which of the Inspiration Suggestions did you choose? What stood out that you'd like to remember?

Go to https://sadnesstojoy.com/forum/21days, and share your thoughts about remembering the happy times from your past.

Day 10 Process Activities

When we read a scripture, devotional, or inspiring quote we tend to think about it for a while. That is called meditating. Meditation is an extension of prayer. The quiet time you spend thinking about what you read or requested is an opportunity for God to speak back to you. It's a chance to ask God what he wants you to do with your prayer requests, or the scripture you read.

Meditation doesn't require you to make funny noises or sit in peculiar positions like you've seen on TV. Just sit in a quiet place and let your mind focus on what you read or requested. What do prayer and meditation look like in your life? If they don't currently exist, what's holding you back?

Day 10 – Prayer Journal

Date:_____

New Prayer Requests	Answered/Outcome

Praise Reports	

Day 10 Reflect Activities

What did you think, talk, and post about today? Were you able to stay focused on the donut (the knowledge you're not alone, you have a God waiting to talk to you and help you), or did you spend the day focused on the hole (the misconception that you're alone, so no one hears you or cares)?

How will you implement what you discovered today to help you find joy?

Was writing down your prayer needs easy or difficult? Was it easier to find prayer needs for yourself or for others? Why do you think that was?

Did writing down the prayer needs of others give you a new perspective on your own needs? How so?

Have you ever prayed or meditated before? If not, why?

What obstacles might you need to overcome to make prayer and meditation a daily habit? How will you overcome them?

Which of the Inspiration Suggestions did you choose? What stood out that you'd like to remember?

Go to https://sadnesstojoy.com/forum/21days, and share your thoughts about prayer and meditation.

Day 11 Process Activities

Everyone is in a different place on this journey. Some are starting from step one, while others are already a thousand steps in. Where you stand on this journey will determine what tools will be most beneficial for you.

Review the list, and remove any tools you won't need. These are things you've already mastered. They aren't a problem for you. For instance, you may be relatively stable and just want to add more joy to your life. If that's the case, you probably won't need the Symptoms Checker.

Now take a second look. Pick out a few you need more immediately. These will be on your toolbelt ready to grab in an instant. The remaining items will be in your toolbox, ready for those special things that come up. Prioritize the items you selected for your Toolbelt. Which three do you need the most and why? These will be the first three you work to develop.

- Creative Avoidance

- Healthy Diet & Exercise

- Identify Triggers

- Laughter

- New View

- Overcoming Obstacles

- Positive Affirmations

- Re-Direction

- Relaxation Techniques

- Serenity Prayer

- Stop, Drop, and Rephrase

- Support Person/Group

- Symptoms Checker

- Worry Willow Tree

Prioritize the items you selected for your Toolbelt. Which three do you need the most and why? These will be the first three you work to develop.

1.

2.

3.

Day 11 – Wellness Progress Report

Listed below are habits which support a joy-filled life. Each night, review the Progress Report, and place a check mark in the box beside each habit you successfully completed that day. You may wish to copy this page first so you will be able to use it repeatedly as you travel this journey.

Habit	Mon	Tues	Wed	Thurs	Fri	Sat	Sun
Count Your Blessings							
Eat Healthy & Drink Plenty of Water							
Set & Follow Plans for Today							
Catch Yourself in Negative Thoughts & Rephrase Them							
Read Scripture or Listen to Inspirational Music							
Spend 30 Minutes Doing Something Physically Active							
Use Positive Self-Talk							
Do Something You Enjoy – That Makes You Smile							
Describe 3 Things Which Made You Happy Today							
Spend Time in Prayer or Meditation							
Practice Relaxation Techniques							

Day 11 – Wellness Goal Sheet

What are your short-term (6-12 months) wellness goals? By what date will you complete them? Use additional sheets if necessary.

Completion Date	Tools to Overcome	Obstacles	Smaller Steps	Goal

Day 11 - Tool Guide

Creative Avoidance – purposely planning an activity to avoid a stressor or trigger

Healthy Diet & Exercise – eating healthy foods, drinking plenty of water, and getting regular exercise as a support to wellness

Identify Triggers – recognition of people, places, things, and events which cause you to be anxious or depressed

Laughter – things that make you smile and laugh such as a joke book, silly videos (YouTube has tons), or a funny movie

New View – looking at your situation from a new perspective, or seeing it from another person's perspective

Overcoming Obstacles – identifying obstacles to wellness habit changes, and planning ways to overcome them

Positive Affirmations – finding & speaking positive things about yourself rather than negative

Re-Direction – distracting yourself from a stressor or trigger for which no plan was made, such as walking away or changing the subject

Relaxation Techniques – music, meditation, soft lighting, hot bath or massage to reduce stress or anxiety

Serenity Prayer – changing what you can (yourself) and accepting what you cannot control (which is everything else)

Stop, Drop, and Rewind – Stop any negative thought, drop any anxiety or emotion it caused, and rewind the thought to make it more positive

Support Person/Group – a compassionate, trustworthy person or group you turn to in a time of need

Symptoms Checker – a place to chart symptoms of depression or anxiety daily

Worry Willow Tree – recognition of something worrisome and a decision tree which determines your action (see sample below)

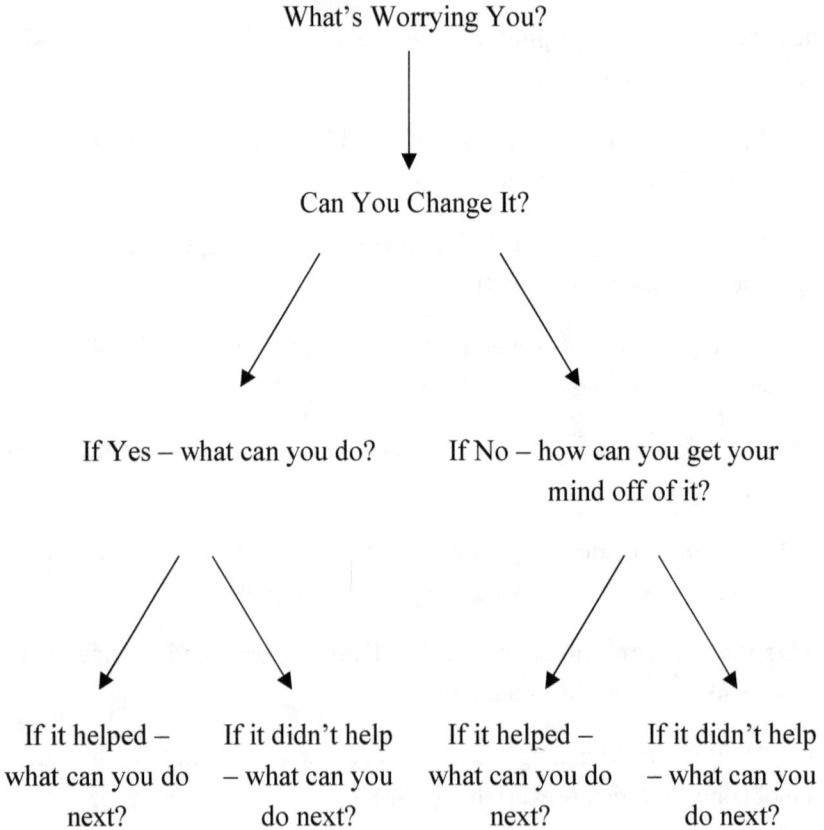

What's Worrying You?

Can You Change It?

If Yes – what can you do?   If No – how can you get your
                                          mind off of it?

If it helped –   If it didn't help   If it helped –   If it didn't help
what can you do   – what can you   what can you do   – what can you
    next?   do next?   next?   do next?

Day 11 – Support Team

Name	Phone, Email, Address
Emergency Health Crisis	911
Suicide Lifeline	1-800-SUICIDE (784-2433)
Medical Professional	
Mental Health Professional	
Spiritual Support Professional	
Family/Friend	
Family/Friend	
Family/Friend	
Family/Friend	
Family/Friend	
Family/Friend	

Day 11 Reflect Activities

What did you think, talk, and post about today? Were you able to stay focused on the donut (there are tools you can use and habits you can develop which will make you feel better), or did you spend the day focused on the hole (you've tried everything and nothing works)?

How will you implement what you discovered today to help you find joy?

What items did you take out of your toolkit? Why?

What items did you move to your toolbelt for immediate access? Why?

How does it feel to know you are learning to use the tools you need to start enjoying your life more?

What were your thoughts as you developed your Wellness Action Plan?

What obstacles might you face in using some of these tools? How will you overcome them?

Which of the Inspiration Suggestions did you choose? What stood out that you'd like to remember?

Go to https://sadnesstojoy.com/forum/21days, and share your thoughts about preparing a Wellness Action Plan.

Day 12 Process Activities

We all have stressors and triggers in our life which cause emotional reactions. The decision to be made is whether it will be a tremor or a full-blown earthquake. What are some things which cause you to react emotionally?

Day 12 – Emotional Explosion/Identify Your Triggers

Date: _____

What happened?	
Who or **What** was the trigger?	
Why did it make me explode?	
How did I respond?	
How could I respond better next time?	

Day 12 Reflect Activities

What did you think, talk, and post about today? Were you able to stay focused on the donut (you can control your emotional explosions), or did you spend the day focused on the hole (some people just know how to push your buttons, you can't help it)?

How will you implement what you discovered today to help you find joy?

Was it easy to identify some of your triggers or did you have a hard time?

What tools did you decide to use? Why?

Which of the Inspiration Suggestions did you choose? What stood out that you'd like to remember?

Go to https://sadnesstojoy.com/forum/21days, and share your thoughts about identifying your triggers and learning to defuse them.

Day 13 Process Activities

It is important for you to self-monitor when it comes to mental health. Track your feelings, and know when you are on overload. How many symptoms are you currently experiencing? Did you realize they might be related? If you have several symptoms listed, how does it make you feel to know you might be suffering from depression? Does it bring relief or fear?

Do you allow your emotions to make decisions for you? Remember to make fact-based decisions. Don't say yes to something begrudgingly. You will only resent doing it on an already overtaxed schedule. Remember to simplify and set boundaries. Get to know yourself, and know when it's time to reach out for help.

If you already suffer from depression, both you and your family need to learn more about it. A strong support team is critical when you are struggling with depression. Do your family and friends know you might be suffering from depression? Don't wait for them to ask if they can help; tell them what they can do to help you.

Day 13 – Depression Awareness

Facts to Remember	Reference Source

Day 13 Reflect Activities

What did you think, talk, and post about today? Were you able to stay focused on the donut (it's okay to say no to something if it's what's best for your own health, knowledge is power and now you have it), or did you spend the day focused on the hole (you have to help everyone even if it's not healthy)?

How will you implement what you discovered today to help you find joy?

How do you feel about the idea of simplifying your life? Are you experiencing anxiety about what others will think if you step away from certain activities? Are you unsure how they will manage without you? What tools can you use to help ease these feelings and do what's best for you?

What symptoms were you able to identify in yourself? Were you surprised to learn you had so many? Did it bring you relief to know there's a name for what you're experiencing?

What did you learn about depression? How can you help yourself or others with this knowledge?

Do you need to go back and re-visit Day 3 and ask for some help?

Which of the Inspiration Suggestions did you choose? What stood out that you'd like to remember?

Go to https://sadnesstojoy.com/forum/21days, and share your thoughts about depression and mental illness.

Day 14 Process Activities

Do you have trouble sleeping? Which of the factors listed may be contributing?

- Medical illness – cold, flu, pain, heartburn, kidney problem, etc.

- Emotional upset – anxiety, depression, worry, anger, etc.

- Prescriptions – read labels carefully, and ask your doctor

- Caffeine overuse or consumption late in the day – coffee, tea, soda Note: Caffeine withdrawal can cause headaches, but stick with it, and they will subside.

- Alcohol consumption

- Eating a heavy meal before bed

- Taking naps

- Exercise or physical activity late in the day

- Electronics – TV, computer, smart phone, video games

- Sleep setting – temperature, strong colors, noise, comfort, etc.

- Irregular sleep schedule – going to bed at different times

What can you do to eliminate, or at least lessen the impact, of whatever factors are affecting your sleep?

Use the links provided to find a solution. Now, plan to implement the changes one at a time to see which one works best for you.

- Centers for Disease Control (CDC) - http://bit.ly/1I50rj7

- Help Guide - http://bit.ly/10jc8kB

- Caring.com - http://bit.ly/1HmQRs9

Did you find anything helpful on these sites? Which strategies can you use to help with your specific sleep problems?

Day 14 - Sleep Tracker – Activity 1

What did you do in the hour leading up to bedtime?

Did you fall asleep easily? Did you take something to help you sleep?

Do you have a sleep routine?

Did you wake up in the middle of the night? Was it difficult to fall back asleep?

What time did you wake up to start your day? By alarm or on your own?

What obstacles did you face? How will you overcome them?

What will you do differently to facilitate better sleep in the future?

Day 14 - Sleep Tracker – Activity 2

Sun					
Sat					
Fri					
Thurs					
Wed					
Tues					
Mon					

Day 14 – Sleep Tracker – Activity 3

Date: _____

What was your goal for last night?

Did you meet it? Why or Why not?

What obstacles did you face? How will you overcome them?

What sleeping tips did you use? How did they work?

How did you feel this morning upon rising?

Day 14 Reflect Activities

What did you think, talk, and post about today? Were you able to stay focused on the donut (you can control how well you sleep, there are things you can do to help), or did you spend the day focused on the hole (no matter what you do, you just can't sleep)?

How will you implement what you discovered today to help you find joy?

What sleep problems have you experienced? What is your typical bedtime routine?

How do you feel about giving up your electronics later in the evening? What activity can you do instead?

How do you feel about giving up caffeine and alcohol later in the day? What can you drink instead?

What obstacles do you think might interfere with your ability to adopt healthier bedtime habits? How will you overcome them?

Which of the Inspiration Suggestions did you choose? What stood out that you'd like to remember?

Go to https://sadnesstojoy.com/forum/21days, and share your thoughts about developing a bedtime routine.

Day 15 Process Activities

Think through things you enjoyed doing when you were younger. Which have you thought about doing lately and talked yourself out of because you're too old or too ... whatever?

Day 15 – Spur of the Moment

Ideas for How to Have Some Fun	Completed

Day 15 Reflect Activities

What did you think, talk, and post about today? Were you able to stay focused on the donut (your life can be fun again) or did you spend the day focused on the hole (you're too old to have fun, what will people think if you do that)?

How will you implement what you discovered today to help you find joy?

What were your thoughts when you read the list of suggestions I made?

What obstacles would you need to overcome to do some of them? How will you overcome them?

How could you be more spontaneous?

Which of the Inspiration Suggestions did you choose? What stood out that you'd like to remember?

Go to   https://sadnesstojoy.com/forum/21days, and share your thoughts about being more spontaneous.

Day 16 Process Activities

Just because your fatigue is normal doesn't mean you should live with it. What can you do today to improve your habits to provide more energy? Pick something from the list, or come up with something on your own. Use the PIRA process to set goals and monitor your progress.

- See your family doctor to rule out any medical cause

- Take up Yoga

- Balance your schedule with your body clock's sleep and wake cycle

- Lose weight

- Eat a healthy breakfast high in fiber, complex carbs, and protein

- Take a break – stand up, stretch, or walk around a bit

- Drink plenty of water

- Unplug or limit mindless electronics - do something mentally active instead

- Increase your B-vitamin intake – it helps fight stress

- Increase your D-vitamin intake – it helps fight depression

Day 16 – Energy Plan

What time of day do you notice a drop in your energy?

What were you doing at the time? Right before?

What was your last meal? How long ago?

What can you do when you notice your energy dropping?

What habit changes can you make to help avoid these energy drops in the future?

Day 16 Reflect Activities

What did you think, talk, and post about today? Were you able to stay focused on the donut (there are things you can do to fight your fatigue), or did you spend the day focused on the hole (you're always tired, it will never change, so why even try)?

How will you implement what you discovered today to help you find joy?

At what time of day does your energy start slipping away? What can you do to counteract that feeling?

Did you notice any patterns to when your fatigue comes on? What can you tweak in your routine to help fight it?

Which of the Inspiration Suggestions did you choose? What stood out that you'd like to remember?

Go to https://sadnesstojoy.com/forum/21days, and share your thoughts about ways to keep your energy level high.

Day 17 Process Activities

How many times have you said to someone, "we need to get together soon," only to say the same thing six months later? Believe me, I get it. We all lead busy lives. But if we don't purposefully plan face-time with others, it simply won't happen. So who do you need to start connecting with in person? How can you make that happen?

Day 17 – Face-Time Plan – Activity 1

How often do you currently have face-time with friends and family outside of work?

What is your Face-Time goal for your first week?

What activity have you chosen? Why?

Who will you meet? Why?

What will you do together? Why did you choose this activity?

What are your feelings about meeting with them face-to-face?

What obstacles do you think you might face? How will you overcome them?

Day 17 – Face-Time Plan – Activity 2

	Sun					
Sun						
Sat						
Fri						
Thurs						
Wed						
Tues						
Mon						

Day 17 – Friendship Circle

Friend	Phone, Email, Address

Things You Can Do Together		
Activity	Cost	Time Needed

Day 17 Reflect Activities

What did you think, talk, and post about today? Were you able to stay focused on the donut (you've got friends, real ones, not just virtual ones), or did you spend the day focused on the hole (no one cares or has time for your problems, you're just a burden on everyone)?

How will you implement what you discovered today to help you find joy?

Think about the five friends you listed earlier whom you haven't seen in six months. What's stopping you from spending face-time with them? What would it take to change that?

Is there someone you need to forgive before you can re-connect? How about someone you need to apologize to before you can re-connect? What's stopping you? Find a way to make this happen sooner rather than later.

How does the idea of meeting with friends make you feel? Why?

What obstacles would you need to overcome to make these interactions more comfortable? How will you overcome them?

Did you have trouble coming up with a list of 5 to 10 friends? What did you decide to do to meet new friends?

Which of the Inspiration Suggestions did you choose? What stood out that you'd like to remember?

Go to https://sadnesstojoy.com/forum/21days, and share your thoughts about spending more face-time with others.

Day 18 Process Activities

Learning something new serves multiple purposes. It gets us out of isolation and connects us with others. It's physically and mentally engaging. And mastering a new skill provides a sense of accomplishment. What's something new you'd like to learn more about?

Day 18 – Short-Term Bucket List

Short-Term Bucket List (6-12 Months)			
Activity	Cost	Time Needed	Completion Date
1			
2			
3			
4			
5			
6			
7			
8			
9			
10			

Day 18 Reflect Activities

What did you think, talk, and post about today? Were you able to stay focused on the donut (learning can be fun, the reward really is worth the risk), or did you spend the day focused on the hole (you're too old to learn new things, people will laugh at you when you don't do it right)?

How will you implement what you discovered today to help you find joy?

Did you have a hard time coming up with 10 things you would enjoy doing? Why do you think that is?

How did you feel about trying something new? What activity did you select to do? Why did you choose that one? Is it comfortable or a challenge?

Did you face any fear about your choice of activity? Did you overcome your fear and take the first step towards making it happen?

Which of the Inspiration Suggestions did you choose? What stood out that you'd like to remember?

Go to https://sadnesstojoy.com/forum/21days, and share your thoughts about trying something new.

Day 19 Process Activities

No one wants to ask for help. Sometimes we don't even know we need it. But kindness is always appreciated. What could someone do to make you feel better in a time of need? If it would help you, it would probably help them as well. What things from the list could you start doing for others? What are some unique ways you could help others based on your strengths?

- Hold the door for someone

- Volunteer at a shelter

- Bake something special for a neighbor or coworker

- Donate gently-used items to a thrift store

- Let someone with fewer items, small children, or elderly go in front of you at the checkout line

- Mow someone's grass who is sick or out of town

- Prepare a meal for someone who is sick or has a family member in the hospital. Better yet, bring a meal to the hospital if their diet allows.

- Let another car cut in front of you in the pick-up line at school

- Visit a sick person in the hospital or elderly person in a care facility

- Pay a compliment to a total stranger

- Smile at someone for no reason

- Volunteer for an organization whose passion you share

Day 19 – Acts of Kindness

Ways I Can Help or Encourage Others	

Day 19 Reflect Activities

What did you think, talk, and post about today? Were you able to stay focused on the donut (you may not be where you want to be, but you're better off than where you were and you're better off than a lot of others), or did you spend the day focused on the hole (you don't have anything to share with others, besides they don't have it as bad as you do, you've got to get better first)?

How will you implement what you discovered today to help you find joy?

Could you relate to the opening story? What would you do if that was you? How would it make you feel?

What are some ways you can think of to help others? What obstacles would need to be overcome for you to go do it?

Which of the Inspiration Suggestions did you choose? What stood out that you'd like to remember?

Go to https://sadnesstojoy.com/forum/21days, and share your thoughts about helping others.

Day 20 Process Activities

Are you currently practicing some form of faith-based worship? If so, does it give you a sense of peace? If not, consider using the seven areas of growth listed above to go deeper. Which area would be the best place for you to start? Why? What could you do in that area to start growing?

- **Desire** – to learn new things about God, to get to know him

- **Study of the Bible** – God's guidebook for our lives

- **Prayer** – a way to communicate with God

- **Worship** – an opportunity to thank God for his blessings

- **Repentance** – sorrow for our sins and attempts to improve

- **Giving** – providing our time, talent, and money for God's church

- **Service** – helping others with our time, talent, and money

Day 20 – Spiritual Growth Plan

Desire - to learn new things about God, to get to know him

Study of the Bible - which is God's guidebook for our lives

Prayer - which is a way to communicate with God

Worship - which is an opportunity to thank God for his blessings

Repentance – sorrow for our sins and attempts to improve

Giving – providing your time, talent, and money for God's church

Service – helping others with your time, talent, and money

Area of Growth	What Will I Do?	When? How Often?

Day 20 Reflect Activities

What did you think, talk, and post about today? Were you able to stay focused on the donut (God has a purpose for your suffering and it's not too late to build a relationship and have Him help you get through it), or did you spend the day focused on the hole (you don't need God, he hasn't helped you so far, why should you trust him now)?

How will you implement what you discovered today to help you find joy?

If you had to assess your status on the spiritual growth journey, which phrase best describes you? Why?

- o   I didn't even know there was a trip planned
- o   I'm just starting out
- o   I'm along for the ride
- o   I'm making steady progress
- o   I'm leading the troops

What would your next step be on this journey?

What obstacles might prevent you from taking that next step? How will you overcome them?

Which of the Inspiration Suggestions did you choose? What stood out that you'd like to remember?

Go to https://sadnesstojoy.com/forum/21days, and share your thoughts about spiritual growth and the habits it requires.

Day 21 Process Activities

I've introduced 21 areas of wellness where positive changes will lead to more joy. How did you do? What grade would you give yourself on your Wellness Journey? Changing habits takes time, so don't get discouraged.

According to our definition in the beginning, joy is a deep feeling or condition of happiness or contentment.[1] My prayer is that you have started developing habits which will help you find happiness and be content as you continue this journey. Thanks for taking it with me.

Wellness Report Card

Area of Wellness	Grade	Area of Wellness	Grade
Count Your Blessings		Identify Your Triggers	
How Food Affects Your Mood		Learn About Depression	
Ask for Help		Get Your Sleep	
Dispute Negative Thoughts		Be Spontaneous	
Have Faith		Energize Yourself	
Get Up and Move		Increase Your Face-Time	
Practice Enjoying Life		Explore New Interests	
Master Your Mind and Habits		Help Others	
Remember Happy Times		Enhance Your Spiritual Life	
Practice Prayer and Meditation		Pick Your Battles	
Create Wellness Habits			

Day 21 – Electronics Challenge

What plans do you have for replacing current electronic activities?

What obstacles will you need to overcome? How will you overcome them?

What are your feelings going into this challenge?

Are you All-In committed?

When will you start the challenge?

When will you finish the challenge?

How will you celebrate when you finish the challenge?

Day 21 – Music Challenge

What plans do you have for finding music you enjoy?

What are some of your choices? From what sources?

What obstacles will you need to overcome? How will you overcome them?

What are your feelings going into this challenge?

Are you All-In committed?

When will you start the challenge? When will you finish the challenge?

How will you celebrate when you finish the challenge?

Day 21 Reflect Activities

What did you think, talk, and post about today? Were you able to stay focused on the donut (you've come so far, you may not be where you want to be yet, but you're not where you started), or did you spend the day focused on the hole (you've tried everything I've said, but nothing worked)?

How will you implement what you discovered today to help you find joy?

What are your thoughts about the Electronics Challenge? Are you up for it?

What obstacles might you face with this Challenge? How will you overcome them?

What are your thoughts about the Music challenge? Are you up for it?

What obstacles might you face with this challenge? How will you overcome them?

Which of the Inspiration Suggestions did you choose? What stood out that you'd like to remember?

Go to https://sadnesstojoy.com/forum/21days, and share your thoughts about your Electronics Challenge or Music Challenge experience.

Notes

Getting Started

1. "Joy", The Free Dictionary by Farlex, accessed October 1, 2016, http://thefreedictionary.com/joy.

Day 1: Count Your Blessings

1. "Need", The Oxford Dictionary, accessed April 15, 2017, https://en.oxforddictionaries.com/definition/need.

2. "Want", The Oxford Dictionary, accessed April 15, 2017, https://en.oxforddictionaries.com/definition/want.

3. "Content", The Free Dictionary by Farlex, accessed October 1, 2016, http://thefreedictionary.com/joy.

4. David Niven, *The 100 Simple Secrets of Happy People: What Scientists Have Learned and How You Can Use It* (New York: Harper Collins, 2006)

Day 2: How Food Affects Your Mood

1. "These 5 Foods and Substances Can Cause Anxiety and Insomnia," Psychology Today, accessed October 6, 2016, http://www.livestrong.com/ article/28412-list-refined-carbs/.

2. "Nutrition," Centers for Disease Control and Prevention, accessed October 12, 2016, https://www.cdc.gov/nutrition/index.html.

3. "Shop the Outer Perimeter to Find Nutrient Dense Food," ShapeFit, accessed October 12, 2016, http://www.shapefit.com/diet/shop-outer-perimeter.html.

4. "Can Food Affect Your Mood," Mercola: Take Control of Your Health, accessed April 18, 2017, http://articles.mercola.com/sites/articles/archive/2014/01/02/food-affects-mood.aspx.

5. My Fitness Pal, accessed April 18, 2017, https://www.myfitnesspal.com/.

Day 4: Dispute Negative Thoughts

1. Lee Strobel, *The Case for Faith: A Journalist Investigates the Toughest Objections to Christianity* (Michigan: Zondervan, 2000).

Day 5: Have Faith

1. Lee Strobel, *The Case for Faith: A Journalist Investigates the Toughest Objections to Christianity* (Michigan: Zondervan, 2000).

2. Lee Strobel, *The Case for Christ: A Journalist's Personal Investigation of the Evidence for Jesus,* (Michigan: Zondervan, 1998).

Day 6: Get Up and Move

1. "The 20 Secrets to a Happy Life," Questia: Trusted Online Research, accessed October 14, 2016, https://www.questia.com/newspaper/1G1-335774685/the-20-secrets-to-a-happy-life-a-10-minute-walk-can.

2. "Unhappy People Watch More Television," Science 2.0, accessed October 14, 2016, http://www.science20.com/news_releases/unhappy_people_watch_more_television.

Day 8: Master Your Mind and Habits

1. "Self-awareness," University of Waterloo Learning Services, accessed October 17, 2016, https://uwaterloo.ca/student-success/sites/ca.student-success/files/uploads/files/TipSheet_SelfAwareness.pdf.

Day 13: Learn About Depression

1. Henry Cloud and John Townsend, *Boundaries: When to Say Yes, How to Say No, To Take Control of Your Life*, (Michigan: Zondervan, 1992).

2. Lysa TerKeurst, *The Best Yes*, (Nashville, Nelson Books, 2014).

3. Victoria Bekiempis, "Nearly 1 in 5 Americans Suffers from Mental Illness Each Year," *Newsweek,* February 28, 2014, accessed November 2, 2016, http://www.newsweek. com/nearly-1-5-americans-suffer-mental-illness-each-year-230608.

Day 14: Get Your Sleep

1. "Insomnia Statistics," The Better Sleep Guide, accessed November 3, 2016, http://www.better-sleep-better-life.com/insomnia-statistics.html.

2. "Are You Getting Enough Sleep," Centers for Disease Control and Prevention, accessed November 3, 2016, https://www.cdc.gov/Features/Sleep/.

Day 16: Energize Yourself

1. "How to Fight Depression Fatigue," Everyday Health, accessed November 6, 2016, http://everydayhealth.com/hs/major-depression-living-well/fight-depression-fatigue/.

2. Stephen Covey, *The Seven Habits of Highly Effective People: Powerful Lessons in Personal Change*, (New York: Free Press, 1989)

Who Am I

I am Human – I make mistakes!
I will accept my mistakes as normal, and
I will focus on my successes, not my failures.

I am Human – I have emotions!
I will experience my emotions, and
I will use self-control in order to respond to facts, not feelings!

I am Human – I have a history!
I will accept both good and bad experiences, and
I will cherish my blessings while using what I learned to help others!

I am Human – I have physical flaws!
I will accept what I see in the mirror as a unique creation, and
I will focus on what I can do instead of what I cannot do.

I am Human – I have strengths and weaknesses!
I will acknowledge I was not made to do everything perfectly, and
I will find ways to use my strengths, while seeking help for my weaknesses.

I am Human – I have unique interests and passions!
I will set aside the expectations of others, and
I will follow my heart, allowing myself to do what brings me joy.

I am Human – I understand right and wrong!
I will do what is right just because it is right, and
I will boldly speak the truth in love to myself, and others, when it is wrong.

I am Human – I am made in the image of God!
I will believe I am a masterpiece, and
I will declare I have a purpose - I am wanted - I am loved!

Vicki Huffman
Copyright © 2015

About the Author

Vicki Huffman is the happily married mother of four children, two natural-born and two God entrusted her to raise for others. She is also the proud grandmother of six. She lives in sunny Florida and lives a truly joy-filled life. However, it hasn't always been that way.

At 14, Vicki was the victim of a violent crime. As a result, she walked away from the God she thought would keep her safe and the faith she'd known her entire life. She wandered through life in a highly functional depressed state for the next 40 years. Until that day!

On October 29, 2014, Vicki suffered a complete emotional breakdown and was hospitalized. She finally admitted she was powerless over her mental illness. She needed help. Following weeks of inpatient and outpatient care, she dedicated her time and energy to starting a new life. A joy-filled life without depression.

Vicki has learned how to leave her life of depression behind and experience a life filled with joy. As a lifelong educator, she knows her purpose in life now is to help teach those who are hurting how they too can lead a joy-filled life.

Follow: @vickihuffman23

Questions: E-mail vicki@sadnesstojoy.com

www.ingramcontent.com/pod-product-compliance
Lightning Source LLC
La Vergne TN
LVHW051503080426
835509LV00017B/1902